The Gifted Child
in Peer Group Perspective

Barry H. Schneider

The Gifted Child in Peer Group Perspective

Springer-Verlag
New York Berlin Heidelberg
London Paris Tokyo

Barry H. Schneider
Child Study Centre
School of Psychology
University of Ottawa
Ottawa, Ontario
Canada K1N 6N5

With 4 Figures

Library of Congress Cataloging-in-Publication Data
Schneider, Barry H.
    The gifted child in peer group perspective.
    Bibliograph: p.
    Includes index.
    1. Gifted children—United States.   2. Age groups—
United States.   3. Interpersonal relations.   I. Title.
HQ773.5.S48   371.95   87-12864

Typeset by Best-set Typesetter Ltd., Quarry Bay, Hong Kong.
Printed and bound by R.R. Donnelley & Sons, Harrisonburg, Virginia.
Printed in the United States of America.

9 8 7 6 5 4 3 2 1

ISBN 0-387-96534-3 Springer-Verlag New York Berlin Heidelberg
ISBN 3-540-96534-3 Springer-Verlag Berlin Heidelberg New York

For Brian and Lauren

Preface
An Applied Psychologist's Initiation
to the Study of Gifted Children

My interest in the subject matter of this book, the peer relations of gifted children, intensified enormously as result of my involvement with one gifted child during my days as a school psychologist. At that time, I served a number of schools in a prosperous suburb. I spent most of my time working with children with behavioral and learning disorders. I received very few requests to assist gifted youngsters and their teachers, perhaps because, at that point, I was not very sensitive to their needs.

One autumn I was involved in something from which I derived a great deal of satisfaction—helping the teachers of a very advanced retarded boy with Down's syndrome maintain himself in a regular first-grade class. In retrospect, the achievements of this student, Jeff, would have justified my calling him exceptionally bright, given the limits of his endowment. I was interrupted from my observation of Jeff's success in class by a phone call from another school, one to which I had not previously been summoned. I was asked to discuss the case of an intellectually gifted child who was bored, moody, difficult, and disliked by those around him.

I drove to Jeremy's school. The lawns were impeccably manicured; the floors gleamed with a fresh coat of wax. Jeremy's parents smiled with as much gleam; his teachers and the school principal were warm and welcoming. The pupils' work was displayed with pride everywhere. In this seemingly ideal educational environment, Jeremy was indeed miserable.

I went on to get to know Jeremy better by means of individual counseling. However, I could not undertake this without coming to grips with my own feelings about devoting time to Jeremy, who, on the surface, already seemed to be in the most helpful of surroundings. A confidant suggested that I should devote at least equal time to Jeremy because he would eventually contribute more to society than Jeff. That argument repulsed me then, as it still does.

My dilemma preoccupied me for several days as I drove from school to school to office. I pondered it as I got stuck in traffic behind some road work. I noticed the sign at the construction site. A new cloverleaf was being built at the cost of $11 million. It would save commuters 5 or 10 minutes a day, depending on exactly how far they lived from the existing interchanges in either direction. I decided that it was sinister to be in a position of deciding whether to spend time attending to the needs of Jeremy or Jeff in a land of plenty where we could be well equipped to take on the challenge of responding to the problems of all children if we truly committed our resources to doing so.

Since that time I have worked with many gifted youngsters, both as clinician and researcher. Through knowing others like Jeremy, as well as gifted children whose backgrounds were totally remote from any stereotype that has emerged in either folklore or professional literature, I have learned that the population of gifted children is highly heterogeneous. They display a wide diversity of gifts and talents and probably the full range of fluctuations in temperament and personality. I have also come to respect the devotion of their parents and teachers.

There are considerable polarities of opinion with regard to what is best for gifted children. Contradictory assumptions about their social behavior pervade the parlance of psychologists, educators, and laypersons. Adherents of various beliefs often defend their positions with energy and passion. Such emotion surely derives from commitment. Equal commitment, and equal passion, accompany beliefs about other types of exceptional children. It is my hope that this book helps reinforce this commitment to gifted children while facilitating more knowledgeable decisions and impressions.

I gratefully acknowledge, first of all, the encouragement of Marjorie Rosenman Clegg, coordinator of the University of Ottawa Research Project on the Social Adjustment of Gifted Children. Two University of Ottawa doctoral candidates, Helen Bienert and Kevin Murphy, collaborated on the Chapters 3 and 4, respectively. Debbie Geller patiently coded the children's stories for Chapter 4. Andrea Piccinin carefully scanned the autobiographies of the eminent that are discussed in Chapter 3. Assistance and encouragement were provided by my secretary, Nicole Widmer. Thanks also to Alastair Younger and Kevin Murphy for their comments on an earlier draft.

Barry H. Schneider

Contents

1
Being Gifted in the Culture of Childhood

This chapter focuses on the theoretical links betwen two psychological constructs that are vitally associated with positive adjustment throughout the lifespan: intelligence and social competence. The intent here is to consider the proposition that individuals endowed with exceptional intellectual abilities should logically be expected to excel in the formation and maintenance of social relationships. Within the context of this deliberation, several conceptualizations of giftedness will be analyzed in terms of their implications for peer relations. The four chapters that follow examine several different types of research that provide information useful in accepting or refuting this proposition.

The Gifted Child as Social Outcast

The prevalence of two types of myth impede objective reasoning about the social relations of the gifted. The first of these is the assumption that bright people are destined to be social outcasts. It is interesting to trace the history of this idea—and, later on, of its converse—in the evolution of beliefs about intelligence and giftedness. This premise may derive from the well-known life stories of famous artists, which have captured the attention of psychoanalysts, biographers, novelists, and the general public. The sufferings, loneliness, and scorn suffered by many upon whom history has bestowed posthumous reverence are well-known. Many believe that these cases are representative of the experience of eminent individuals. The lives of prominent people in other walks of life have received less attention. The social and emotional world of the gifted scientist, statesman, or carpenter may or may not be as troubled. In any event, the products of their gifts inherently bear fewer scars of any loneliness or emotional pain. Therefore, if they do suffer from isolation—or derive inspiration from it—they are more likely to do so privately. Loneliness is more readily ascribed to a great painting than to a master craftsman's furniture.

Although they are not as widely known, similar case studies have been conducted with young children. For example, Feldman (1982) followed 69 "Quiz Kids" who participated in a radio quiz show for children in the 1940s into adolescence and adulthood. She concluded that

...those of us who became national figures at an early age were subjected to a constant barrage of attention....The social penalties were exacerbated by our being younger, smaller and less physically coordinated than our classmates. The problem became most severe during adolescence, when identity formation and peer relationships became all-important. The way each of us handled our situation depended, in the final analysis, upon the personal baggage we carried to it. No doubt some of us were hypersensitive; I'm sure I was. (Feldman, 1982, p. 360)

Some of the "Quiz Kids" also developed a deep distaste for their own talents and an overmastering need to be ordinary. This is no less tragic an ending to the story.

Hollingworth's (1942) study of children with IQs over 180 is a classic in the literature on gifted children. The bright, young child was portrayed therein as being basically friendly but tending to play alone. An early interest in reading was said to heighten this isolation—or, perhaps, result from it. This isolated play was ascribed to the fact that bright children are far more mature both physically and mentally than other children. It is interesting to note that conceptions of giftedness at that time almost always included physical characteristics.

Writing on behalf of gifted youth, David Cooke, a 15-year-old freshman at Midland Park (New Jersey) High School submitted an essay on the social life of gifted children to the Johns Hopkins University Center for the Advancement of Academically Talented Youth. It was reprinted in the New York Times on June 24, 1985, and ended as follows:

Loneliness is the price I seem to pay for my gifts. I have never had enough close friends who think as I do. In early childhood, I even created an imaginary playmate to try to cope with my loneliness. I do have several wonderful friends, extraordinarily gifted in math and other subjects. Sadly, I sense that they, too, are outsiders who spend a lot of time locked alone in their rooms. They don't go often to school dances, are rarely or never invited to parties and stay away from school sports events because they are different from the crowd.

We are not sick, we are not neurotic. We are just different, lonely and acutely aware and regretful of our outsider status.

Interestingly, there are many reports of gifted children resorting to the company of imaginary playmates to escape their painful feelings of solitude. However, not all researchers have found that the imaginary companion phenomenon is associated with higher levels of intelligence (Manosevitz, Fling, & Prentice, 1977).

A pamphlet on counseling gifted children distributed by the U.S. National Association for Gifted Children (Schmitz & Galbraith, 1985) begins by reminding the reader that *not all* gifted children need counseling (emphasis added). Janos, Marwood, and Robinson (1985) found that basic textbooks on giftedness often include specific social behavior problems among the characteristics that are said to typify bright children. In 1985, the American Psychological Association (APA) published a comprehensive and well-documented reader on the gifted and talented (Horowitz & O'Brien, 1985); this attention by the APA constituted in itself a landmark contribution to the field. The opening chapter bore the title "The Gifted in Our Midst: By Their Divine Deeds, *Neuroses*, and mental Test Scores We Have Known Them" (emphasis added; Grinder, 1985). It is hard to dispute the fact that the neuroses of the gifted are indeed well-known.

The Pervasive Benign Light of Intelligence

The opposite assumption—that persons who achieve high IQs are destined to succeed in all areas of functioning—is not without its adherents. This presupposal is probably the legacy of a generation of psychologists who enshrined the IQ construct on a pedestal higher than is merited by its undeniable validity and utility. Many members of that generation considered intelligence a one-dimensional construct. The one single dimension of ability was presumed to apply to virtually all types of activities. Social relations were but one more example of the areas in which the intelligent were sure to display the ubiquitous benefits of high IQ.

Early case studies, especially those by Terman (1925) provided some evidence for this contention, which is now dubbed "the Terman myth." Terman's works were landmarks in the field. In 1959, three years after his death, Terman was ranked third in a list of the 10 most outstanding psychologists in American history by the APA (Sattler, 1982). Terman contended that gifted children excelled on virtually all traits of personality, intellect, and character. He vigorously refuted the notion that talent in the intellectual sphere was counterbalanced by deficits in other areas. In fact, the gifted children in Terman's sample had less interest than nongifted peers in social activities. Terman interpreted even this finding as a further indication of the tendency of the gifted to excel at all things: he attributed it to their self-reliance. He also carefully noted that the play of the gifted child, as measured by age norms for factual information about games, was highly advanced. His measures of "character"—on which gifted students scored higher than controls in every section—included such socially relevant aspects as emotional stability an "social attitudes." He collected teacher ratings of five social traits for gifted and control subjects: leadership, sensitivity to approval, popularity, freedom from vanity, and fondness for large groups. While the gifted students were rated somewhat higher than controls on all of these, the difference was only substantial[1] for

---

[1] Terman did not use statistical tests of significance as we now know them. Furthermore, many of his interpretations were clearly colored by his previous conclusion that "gifted children at all ages are less likely than controls to overstate their knowledge." (Terman, 1925, p. 425)

leadership (see following discussion of other early leadership studies). The gifted child's excellence in leadership was confirmed in a follow-up study, which indicated that bright children were frequently elected to class honors although they were often the youngest children in the class. While noting the superiority of the gifted children in virtually all traits, Terman carefully reminded the reader that these were *average* differences and that there were marked fluctuations within the gifted child population (as with the controls; Terman & Oden, 1959). Rarely highlighted in subsequent literature, and not woven into the fabric of the "Terman myth," was his observation that those with the highest IQs (170 or above) among the sample of gifted children tended to have more difficulties of social relations than the moderately gifted (Burks, Jensen, & Terman, 1930; Janos, 1983; Terman, 1925). More will be said about this distinction in Chapter 2.

Single-factor models of intelligence are nearing extinction in the theoretical writings on the subject. However, tests based on one-factor conceptions of IQ have hardly disappeared from the market, including instruments used for the identification of gifted pupils in many school districts. Exaggerated assumptions about IQ have penetrated the belief systems of many.

Not all early theories of intelligence implied the existence of one single factor. In contrast with the first simple tests of "intelligence," Kraeplin intended to measure a wide variety of intellectual tasks representative of tasks needed in everyday life (Wolf, 1973). Binet's reflections on the nature of intelligence indicate the prominent role he assigned to judgment. "In intelligence there is a fundamental faculty...that faculty is judgment, otherwise called good sense, practical sense, initiative, the faculty of adapting oneself to circumstances (Binet & Simon, 1973, p. 42). Binet considered it crucial that the assessment of intelligence comprise these socially relevant skills as well as a variety of other capacities: memory, coordination, visual judgment, imagination, attention (Wolf, 1983).

In later intelligence scales, such as Wechsler's, judgment in social situations is considered one of the subcomponents of global IQ. This ability is typically measured by asking the subjects what they would do in a series of social problem situations. The central role of social judgment is emphasized to at least some degree in most prevailing theories of intelligence.

Abroms (1985) outlines a number of cognitive skills that have been associated with social competence in the more recent literature and which have served as cornerstones for many social skills training programs. She begins this presentation with a discussion of social perception, that is, the ability to accurately interpret the verbal and (especially) nonverbal cues and signals sent by the other parties in a social transaction.

The process of social perspective taking is considered by many to be fundamental to the emergence of mature social relationships. This skill is an extension to the interpersonal sphere of Piaget's more cognitive notion of perspective taking. It involves the understanding of the thinking of the other individual or individuals in a social situation. It is important not only to appreciate the perspective of the other but to coordinate the understanding of the other's vantage point with one's own thinking (Feffer, 1970; Flavell, 1968). Empathy is a related construct.

The process of solving social problems has captured the attention of both clinical and developmental psychologists. Three types of problem-solving skills were included in Spivack and Shure's (1974) well-known social skills training program intended for use in regular kindergartens and in many subsequent programs. The first skill is alternative solutions thinking, the ability to conceive of a number of different solutions to a problematic social dilemma. Consequential thinking is the logical next step; this refers to the ability to predict the probable consequences of a social act. The third skill area emphasized is means–end thinking, the ability to conceptualize the steps needed to get to a social goal. It has often been found that children with behavior disorders and peer relations problems are deficient in these and other related problem-solving abilities (e.g., Asarnow & Callan, 1985; Camp, 1977).

Piaget (1981) included the capacity for self-estimation in his discussion of the impact of intelligence on affectivity. This capacity to externally and objectively reflect upon one's own behavior may be instrumental in regulating one's interpersonal actions and achieving desired change. Meichenbaum (1975) emphasized the process of self-evaluation, the ability to reflect upon one's social behavior. The "superordinate processes regulating task analysis and self-management of problem-solving behavior" are central in the conception of giftedness expounded by Jackson and Butterfeld (1986).

Abroms (1985) argues that these social components should be considered a distinct type of intelligence and that exceptional talent in this area should be considered a distinct type of giftedness. She notes that Freud implied a specific skill in knowing how to deal with people; he called those with this gift *Menschenkinder*. Citing studies by Rubin (1973) as well as Van Lieshout, Leckie, and Van Sonsbeek (1973), Abroms (1985) notes that correlations between "social intelligence" and overall IQ have been found to be low or moderate. This provides empirical support for regarding social intelligence as somewhat distinct from other areas of intellect. Similarly, interpersonal ability is considered one of seven independent forms of intelligence within Gardner's theory of multiple intelligences (Gardner, 1983; Walters & Gardner, 1986). Gardner identifies social perception as the "core" of this component of intellect, especially "the ability to notice and make distinctions among other individuals, and, in particular, among their moods, temperaments, motivations, and intentions" (Gardner, 1983, p. 239). However, he is sensitive to a well-documented and important reality: Enhanced social cognition is not always manifest in behavior and therefore not always distinguishable by peers. As Gardner puts it, "Forms of personal intelligences, no less than forms of other intelligences, can misfire or fail in their intent, and 'know-that' does not readily or reliably translate into 'know-how'" (Gardner, 1983, p. 241).

The implications of separating these social-cognitive capabilities from other intellectual abilities that are less directly related to interpersonal relations are not clear. Presumably, individuals endowed with social giftedness should display exemplary peer relations. At first glance, there would not be a strong theoretical basis for a connection between the nonsocial aspects of intelligence and observable interpersonal skill. However, even "schoolhouse" intellect (see following discussion)—the abilities needed to succeed in language arts, mathematics, and so on, may not be without implications for peer relations. Over the course of childhood, children spend many thousands of hours in academic lessons. While there may be little direct social contact between peers during academic lessons (Loranger, 1984), it is clear that children's experiences of success and failure in school occur in the presence of the peer group. Since these experiences are repeated almost daily throughout childhood, it is unlikely that peers would have no reaction to the gifted youngster's scholastic prowess. Their responses might range from genuine admiration, to grudging admiration, to envious scorn. Also, these experiences of success may generate a sense of self-confidence, or perhaps overconfidence, that might spill over to other areas of social behavior.

While there are compelling reasons to consider each of the social-cognitive skills discussed above as facilitators of social relations, it is not inconceivable that, at least in certain circumstances, they are drawbacks. Bright children may be a potentially valuable resource to their peers. They know the social norms and may be keen observers and interpreters of the social environment. However, some observers of group process (see following discussion) do not consider knowledge as an unambiguous asset. This opinion is shared by most members of at least one eighth-grade class in Ottawa, in which a rather good-natured boy who always has the right information is incessantly taunted as a "llatiwonk" ("knowitall" spelled backward). This youngster is in fact not at all intrusive in his supply of facts and explanations.

While social sensitivity, empathy, and understanding the thinking of others are clearly desirable characteristics, they can, after a point, become impediments. Higher levels of empathy can lead to distress and indecision (Savage, 1985). Self-evaluation, if carried to excess, can lead to self-reproach, hesitation, and unreasonable standards for oneself and others.

The generation of alternative solutions is only an asset to peer relations in social systems that are prepared to accept the existence of alternative ways of thinking and acting. On the Wechsler scales, the Comprehension items previously mentioned (i.e., those that measure judgment in social situations) usually have only one correct solution, although there is sometimes partial credit for others. Piaget's study of the child's thinking about rules of a game (Piaget, 1932), extended by Kohlberg to the interpersonal domain (Kohlberg, 1969), indicates that the young child considers the rules as rigid, inflexible, inherent in the situation, and externally imposed. Alternative solutions can be seen as challenges to explicit or implicit social rules, values, or norms.

Intelligence, Leadership, and Role Differentiation in Small Groups

Psychologists and sociologists in the first half of the 20th century devoted much attention to the characteristics of the effective leader. This interest was surely spurred by the political climate of the times. There were sweeping upheavals in many countries. Charismatic leaders emerged, triumphed, and were surrounded by flocks of ardent followers. In addition, the military required knowledge that might lead to enhanced leadership, especially in emergency situations.

A comprehensive review of this literature was conducted shortly after the World War II (Stogdill, 1948). Summarizing a half century of research, Stogdill concluded that high intelligence was associated with leadership in 23 of the 29 (child and adult) studies that had investigated both these variables. Futhermore, these and other studies demonstrated that several other intellective variables—insight, knowledge, judgment—were associated with attainment of the leadership role. These dimensions fell outside the perimeter of the rather narrow notions of intelligence that prevailed at the time. However, they are included in some modern conceptualizations of giftedness, which will be discussed shortly.

Some limits on the relation between intelligence and leadership had become apparent in the research. Five studies had replicated Hollingworth's (1942) finding that the gifted were not well regarded in situations where there was a very large discrepancy between their IQs and those of their peers. Stogdill carefully noted that he was reviewing the literature on leadership not popularity. However, very high correlations were found between leadership and popularity in most of the studies. Therefore, the two constructs were regarded as close but not synonymous.

Stogdill and his contemporaries recognized a number of factors aside from intelligence that were associated with leadership. among these were persistence and initiative, qualities that would be seen a quarter century later as important in the emergence of gifted behaviors (see following discussion of Renzulli's 1978, 1986, model). On the other hand, "stability of mood" had also been found crucial in the behavior of leaders. This dimension has proven troublesome for many gifted artists and writers.

Postwar research added further qualifications to the reckoning of the benefits of intelligence in small-group functioning. In an imaginative laboratory study conducted in the 1950s, Guetzkow (1968) extended Leavitt's (1951) classic study of the processes of communication in small groups. In the task presented by Leavitt and Guetzkow, groups of five university undergraduates were seated around a table, separated by partitions that prevented them from seeing each other while performing the problem-solving tasks. Each of the five was given five bits of information out of a standard set of six. Their task was to determine which bit of information was held in common and report it to the experimenter. During the tasks, subjects communicated with each other by passing notes to each other through slots in the partitions. The experimenters could easily adjust the apparatus to allow each subject to communicate only with an adjacent subject, with any other subject, or only with a person at the "hub."

In Guetzkow's (1968) extension of this well-known study, he diminished the importance of the task itself, in order to emphasize the group's structuring and planning activities. The participants discussed the organization and planning of the tasks for several minutes between trials. He divided the 380 subjects into quintiles by IQ (the upper quintile of IQ among university undergraduates in 1956 probably approached an IQ level that many educators would consider in the identification of giftedness). Each group was composed of one member of each IQ quintile. In *groups that successfully organized themselves*, the member with the highest IQ tended to occupy the most crucial role, "keyman." However, about half the groups failed to organize by interlocking their roles. Guetzkow's discussion questions the impact of intelligence in the facilitation of group organization and planning, even in task-oriented groups. Correlations between IQ and his quantitative measures of group planning and process approached zero. Of course, Guetzkow's methodology included many features of studies conducted at that time, which modern social psychologists sharply decry—the overreliance on male undergraduates as representatives of the population, the contrived nature of the task, and random nature of the associations between the participants. However, it ws significant in that it may have helped motivate scholars to look beyond IQ in examining the correlates of leadership.

In the heyday of encounter groups, clinicians studying the differentiation of group roles developed a number of useful distinctions that likely apply to the role of many gifted children and adults in small groups. The roles of information provider and evaluator of ideas are usually included in their taxonomies (e.g., Lifton, 1972). When executed in ways that are pertinent and nondominating, these roles were seen as facilitative of the group process. However, the giver of unwanted advice, as well as the group member who asserted superior status, was considered an obstacle.

Intelligence, Social Competence, and the Prediction of Adult Mental Health

Both intelligence and social competence have been widely validated as part of the equipment useful in overcoming life's obstacles and succeeding in one's endeavors. For example, both variables have some connection with adult mental illness and resistance to it (Cowen, Pederson, Babijian, Izzo, & Trost, 1973; Kohlberg, LaCrosse, & Ricks, 1972; Parker & Asher, 1986). Thus, one might predict that children endowed with high levels of both would become superpersons. However, most psychological research on the prediction of adult mental health has not specifically looked at the extreme upper limits of the IQ range. This is especially the case for the large-scale epidemiological studies that have graphically documented the relation between both childhood social competence and intelligence and psychological adjustment in later life.

In statistical terms, there are little data available that permit the assumption that the relationship between IQ and later socioemotional adjustment is a linear one. In addition, the interactive effects of intelligence and social competence have not often been analyzed statistically in epidemiological studies designed to illuminate the effects of stress and processes of coping, although, presumably, these data are available. Therefore, the fact that intelligence and later adjustment are interrelated *for the entire population* does not necessary mean that individuals with the highest IQs will achieve higher levels of adaptation in life. As discussed more fully in Chapters 2 and 5, some sources suggest that there may be a maximal IQ level above which adaptation and coping do not appear to be facilitated by intellectual abilities. Furthermore, there are very few longitudinal studies that have systematically followed children who display keen intellectual abilities but who lack social skills. Do these children fare any better than their socially unskilled counterparts of average intellectual ability?   .

Motivation and Creativity in Peer Relations Perspective

Most recent authorities have emphasized the need to go beyond IQ in our understanding of giftedness (e.g., Sternberg & Davidson, 1986). The best known of these more comprehensive conceptions is Renzulli's (1978, 1986) triad model. Renzulli speaks of gifted behaviors rather than gifted individuals. He proceeds to describe three variables that, in his view, increase the likelihood of an individual displaying gifted behaviors. The first of Renzulli's three clusters is above-average intellectual ability. He notes that this may be general or specific intellectual ability. There are two other clusters that must also be in evidence. The first is task commitment—

the tendency to confidently pursue an endeavour steadily enough to achieve excellence. The final cluster is creativity, which is identified with such descriptors as "originality of thought," "openness to experience," and "curious, speculative, and adventurous" (Renzulli, 1986, p. 75).

Renzulli (1986) refers to the intellectual talents that can be discovered by means of contemporary measures of intelligence as "schoolhouse giftedness" and feels compelled to discuss the limits of their validity in predicting the emergence of gifted behaviors. Ironically, Binet's original conceptualization of intelligence clearly accentuated components of attentiveness and inventiveness (Wolf, 1973). In our current practice, we have deeply buried the richness of models of intelligence that were well explicated almost a century ago and that could have been extremely useful. Perhaps we shall make better use of the more comprehensive models of intelligence that are increasingly evident in the contemporary literature.

What implications might heightened task commitment and creativity have for peer relations? Peers may well respect well-motivated individuals who are endowed with the stick-to-itiveness needed to get things done. Their creative accomplishments may be the focus of admiration. The very belief in the pursuit of one's own goals may in itself be considered psychologically adaptive. Such individuals feel that their own effort actively helps determine their outcome in life. This psychological dimension is known as *locus of control*. It has been extensively studied and found to relate to several indices of positive social adjustment (Gilmour, 1978; Lefcourt, 1982). Individuals who think this way are known to possess a number of characteristics that should make them more popular with peers. They are more empathic (Thomson-Roundtree, Caldwell, & Webb, 1981), react better in times of stress (Lefcourt, 1982), and are less aggressive in their responses (Bhatia & Golin, 1978). Children who are convinced of the value of their own efforts may see more value in actively seeking the company of others. There is every reason to believe that children who take the initiative in joining peer groups will achieve greater peer acceptance, provided their group entry strategies are socially competent (Dodge, Schlundt, Schocken, & Delugach, 1983; Putallaz, 1983). Cohen and Oden (1974) studied the relationship between children's creativity and locus of control. Their findings were somewhat complex. The correspondence of creativity and locus of control scores depended on the age and sex of the subjects. Older creative children and younger creative girls were external in their locus of control orientation (i.e., they believed that their outcomes depended on their actions).

On the other hand, truly creative, committed individuals may, at certain times and to varying degrees, have to withdraw from social interaction in order to achieve their goals. Reflections on the creative process often indicate that the creative work becomes the overriding concern of the creator. Ties with family members and intimate friends may or may not be impaired as result. However, these reflections leave no doubt that many highly creative people have little time for social life. Thomas Wolfe's description of the production of a novel is not atypical:

I reached that state of naked need and utter isolation that every artist has got to meet and conquer if he is to survive at all. ...I had committed my life and my integrity so irrevocably to this struggle that I must conquer now or be destroyed. I was alone with my own work, and now I knew that I had to be alone with it...I had to get it out of me somehow. (Wolfe, 1952, p. 193)

A related image is conveyed in psychoanalytic portraits of the lives of creative painters and sculptors. Psychodynamically oriented writers have regarded the relationship between artists and the objects they create as an expression of the artists' "love affair with the world." The lives of Michelangelo and David are frequently cited as examples (Weissman, 1971; see also Chapter 3 here for studies of contemporary artists). This love affair has its beginnings in early childhood. The potential for this love affair derives from the ability to be uncommonly flexible in emotional investment (cathexis), a "unique capacity to supplant personal objects with collective alternates. These capacities imply a greater than average expandability for and expendability of object relationships" (Greenacre, 1957 cited in Weissman, 1971).

Some theorists operate on the assumption that creative behavior will not be reinforced by a child's peer group (Barron, 1965). They assume that the independent, determined, sensitive ways of creative children will be regarded as "wild," "naughty," or "crazy" by other children (e.g., Torrance, 1960). Anecdotal data are usually offered in support of this position. Many of the classic early case studies of creative genius revealed that youngsters with the seeds of eminence were often considered stupid, because they either did not pay attention to what was being taught in school, or did not in fact understand the content of the prescribed curriculum. Specific examples include the early school careers of Pestalozzi, Wellington, Burns, Balzac, Humboldt, Boccaccio, and Newton. Their apparent feeblemindedness often earned them the scorn of peers as well as adults (Lombroso, 1891).

Because of the presumed hostility of peers, one of the conditions sometimes seen as essential for the emergence of creativity is a lowered level of susceptibility to social evaluative cues. Heilbrun (1971) implicated the mother's child-rearing practices in the development of susceptibility to social evaluation. He found that a maternal style of high control and low nurturance was linked with both low creativity and heightened susceptibility to evaluative influence. More recent trends in developmental psychology emphasize the bidirectional interpretation of such data. A child who is responsive to social evaluation may well reinforce a mother's controlling behaviors, although probably not her nurturance. Contemporary critics might also decry the fact that only maternal behavior was studied, aggravating child psychology's propensity to blame mothers for all evils of their children. The ability and courage to maintain a degree of independence from peer group opinion is emphasized here as instrumental in the development of creativity. The same type of independence has emerged as an aspect of general emotional adjustment in the personality theory expounded by Albert Ellis (1975).

Getzels and Jackson (1962) urged educators to be tolerant of the solitude needed by creative children. They contended (p. 126) that it is sometimes necessary to put aside modern education's emphasis on group dynamics and peer group experience. However, they made a distinction between healthy solitude and morbid withdrawal, a distinction not as apparent in the reflections of many creative artists.

At certain periods in history, isolation was also seen as fundamental in the emergence of aspects of giftedness other than creativity. Yoder (1894), a scholar who examined the boyhoods of great men, considered it important for bright children to get to know themselves. He saw solitude, in moderation, as essential for such self-knowledge and decried the fact that

...children today are hustled hither and thither from school to society, from church to athletics; every child belongs to a long list of clubs, societies, and fraternities even—there is no time for the child. He knows his playmates better than himself, probably has spent more time, because of favorable opportunity, in studying his friends than he has in studying himself. (Yoder, 1894, p. 154)

Although there are contemporary psychologists and educators who similarly decry the degree of pressure placed on children, especially gifted children, few would subscribe to Yoder's prescription of solitude.

Depression and melancholia have often been thought of as part of the creative process. Andreasen and Canter (1975) traced the evolution of these ideas. Creativity was associated with both melancholia and epilepsy by the ancient Greeks. Aristotle observed that "those who have been eminent in philosophy, politics, poetry and the arts have all had tendencies toward melancholia" (cited in Andreasen & Canter, 1975, p. 196). After a dormant period during the Middle Ages, renewed interest in this connection ensued the rekindled interest in individuality during the Renaissance, 18th, and 19th centuries. If depression in fact accompanies creativity, creativity may inhibit peer acceptance. In his social interaction model of depression, Coyne (1976) emphasized the negative feelings that the interpersonal behavior of the depressed person generates in others. Recent research by Peterson and her colleagues suggests that children also react negatively to the behavior of depressed peers (Peterson, Mullins, & Ridley-Johnson, 1985).

The notion that insanity is associated with creativity has emerged repeatedly throughout history. Such references usually pertain to adults. It has generally been assumed that early signs of eminence are evident in childhood. Beyond that, the classics provide conflicting views of the psychological implications of such precocity. There are some indications that genius and insanity were thought to have common roots in childhood:

This precocity is morbid and atavistic; it may be observed among all savages. The proverb "A man who has genius at five is mad at fifteen" is often verified in asylums. The children of the insane are often precocious. Savage knew an insane woman whose children could play classical music before the age of six, and other children who at a tender age displayed the passions of grown men. Among the children of the insane are often revealed aptitudes and tastes—chiefly for music, the arts, and mathematics—which are not usually found in other children. (Lombroso, 1891, p. 16)

Lombroso's view that psychological disorders were rampant among the highly intelligent was echoed by Ellis (1904), who studied over 1,000 eminent British personalities. Based on hundreds of case studies, Lombroso also concluded that famous men tended not to procreate.

Lombroso's contemporary, Frances Galton, arrived at a totally diametric conclusion. He found that genius was basically hereditary in origin (Galton, 1962). The parents of the eminent men he studied seem as hyperadjusted as the sons. Galton was well aware of Lombroso's contention that creativity was associated with insanity and vigorously disputed it. A revealing critique of Galton's work (Gould, 1981) outlines how these views have been used to support doctrines of racial supremacy. (Gould also presents a number of telling criticisms of the revered Terman studies, previously discussed.)

Role of the Peer Group

In the preceding discussion, the focus has been on the impact of giftedness on a person's social relations. Too little attention has been devoted by theorists and researchers to characteristics of the peer group. As is the case for any minority, the social acceptance of the gifted depends in part on the readiness in society to accept, even appreciate, their unique attributes.

The behavior of nations may be taken as an indication of society's attitude toward the gifted. Many sources point out the increased concern for the education of the gifted in the United States that followed the Soviet Union's dramatic success in launching Sputnik into outer space in 1957 (e.g., Fox & Washington, 1985; Gruber, 1985). Within the recent memory of that generation, one of the soundest electoral trouncings was suffered by Adlai Stevenson; his intellectual pursuits are often cited as at the partial reason for his humiliating failure in this election. During his 1956 presidential campaign, the size of the "egghead vote" and the specter of the "egghead menace" were issues that had penerated everyday conversations about political life (Muller, 1967, p. 189). A few years after Sputnik, an American vice-president, Spiro Agnew was quoted in the press as decrying the influence of an "effete corps of impudent snobs who characterize themselves as intellectuals." (As Agnew, 1970) Envious of the Russian space achievements, North American society was ready to reassess its attitude toward giftedness but perhaps not toward the gifted.

Parallel experiences in other societies are not unknown. One of the best-educated individuals to serve in political office is Israel's former foreign minister, Abba Eban, an acknowledged linguist and scholar of ancient civilizations. Despite his oratory skill and diplomatic acumen, Eban did not get very far in Israeli politics. His biographer, Robert St. John, recalled the following comments, which appeared in an English–Jewish publication shortly after Eban's television appearance in 1959:

Mr. Abba Eban in particular was guilty of speaking over the heads of his viewers. Outstanding as an orator, he was equally at home with the television cameras, but here he was not speaking to the world's diplomats and here his fluency, precision and logic would have little impact on an audience nurtured on "Cheyenne" and "Wagon Train." (St. John, 1973, p. 345)

Eban's erudite manner was also satirized by cartoonists and columnists in the Israeli press.

While we have these and other examples of the adult world's attitudes toward the gifted minority, the place of giftedness in the culture of children is not well documented beyond the popular assumption (see preceding discussion) that gifted children are ill treated. The attitudes of peer toward gifted children are discussed later in this volume.

Age Differences in the Social Adjustment of the Gifted

Janos and Robinson (1985) correctly point out that there is usually considerable continuity in the personal traits of eminent individuals from childhood into adult life. Nevertheless, many retrospective accounts of the lives of the gifted relate a difficult period for peer relations. The precise ages during which social difficulties intensified vary enormously. Nevertheless, there are several reasons to expect that the social adjustment and peer acceptance of the gifted might vary with age.

One possible source of age differences is environmental. The social circle of preschoolers is usually limited to their immediate neighborhood. Therefore, a gifted preschooler will probably have playmates who represent many levels of intellect and creativity. Similarly, bright children in elementary school usually associate with classmates of all interests and proclivities. At this age, they have little opportunity to choose their educational environments. Therefore, they are basically unable to select peers who share their talents and interests. By adolescence and in adulthood, on the other hand, there are more options available in the choice of school subjects, extracurricular activities, and later on, careers and communities. These choices make it much more possible to determine one's own peer group. Thus, a gifted person could by this point succeed in totally avoiding a peer group that devalued his or her interests and more readily gravitate toward more compatible and more sympathetic social surroundings.

On the other hand, adolescence is also a time when, as previously noted, considerations of peer group identity reach the fore. There is often a need to conform in order to achieve identity with the peer group. Thus, the special attributes of the gifted may be less appreciated by themselves and others.

There may be other age differences in the peer group's tolerance for diversity and in its appreciation of creativity and intellect. As previously discussed, the young child may not have the cognitive apparatus to appreciate a variety of perspectives. However, the young child may not yet have a crystallized set of stereotypes about such minorities as the gifted, or a well-ingrained hierarchy of acceptable and unacceptable personal characteristics for potential associates and friends.

Gifted children are, at least in theory, likely to profit from experience (see the preceding discussion of self-evaluation). This would lead us to predict that, over time, they would learn to modulate the ways in which they express their giftedness, to share the vernacular of the peer group. Hopefully, this familiarity with the ways of the nongifted majority does not lead to the renunciation of gifted behavior.

Considerable attention has been devoted recently to society's suppression of the talents of females. This literature will be remembered, but not reviewed, here. However, sex differences as well as age differences will be considered in succeeding chapters.

Organization of this Book

From this point, the focus on giftedness in childhood as opposed to adolescence or adulthood sharpens. Several different methods of analysis are utilized in this probe. Most of the remaining chapters are devoted to an examination of the evidence pertaining to the ideas raised in this chapter.

Chapter 2 is a survey of empirical research on the peer acceptance of bright children. In order to describe that body of knowledge and adequately portray both its strengths and shortcomings, it will be necessary to share with the reader some of the challenges inherent in conducting empirical studies with gifted children. These studies are useful in appreciating the social status of those with the potential for gifted behavior. A complementary method is employed in Chapter 3, in which the childhood social relations of eminent individuals are examined retrospectively. This technique has the advantage of permitting a focus on those who have in fact cultivated their potential for giftedness sufficiently for public attention to be drawn to their accomplishments. Hopefully, this more subjective technique captures the special circumstances and talents that facilitate the emergence of gifted behavior in individuals endowed with such potential.

There has been too little attention to the attitudes of society toward the gifted and the determinants of those attitudes. Chapter 4 considers one possible source of children's impressions of brightness: the portrayal of brightness in children's literature.

At the same time, the social relations of the gifted—and their psychological consequences—should not be thought of as the simple reflection of the behavior of peers. In Chapter 5, the focus shifts to the gifted child's internalization of peer experience. Much of that chapter is devoted to research on the social self-concepts of gifted children.

Chapter 6 profiles the lives and problems of gifted children who have been referred for psychological evaluation because of peer relations difficulties. The influence of brightness on these children's maladjustment is contemplated.

The final chapter, Chapter 7, is devoted to the educational implications of the conclusions drawn throughout this book. Suggestions regarding the counseling and education of gifted children are preceded by a brief review of research documenting the impact of special programming on the social development of gifted children.

In the next six chapters, we shall embark on several different tacks en route to a comprehensive, documented portrayal of the peer relations and psychosocial adjustment of the young gifted in our midst. In describing each of these research approaches, the intent is to share with the reader not only the inferences the researchers have drawn but the methods used to reach them. This should provide not only a summary of what is known about the social development of gifted children but also a feeling for the level of confidence appropriate for each conclusion.

References

Abroms, K.I. (1985). Social giftedness and its relationship with intellectual giftedness. In J. Freeman (Ed.), *The psychology of gifted children* (pp. 201–218). Chichester, England: Wiley.

Andreasen, N.C. & Canter, A. (1975). Genius and insanity revisited: Psychiatric symptoms and family history in creative writers. In R. Wirt, G. Winokur, and M. Roff (Eds.), *Life history research in psychopathology* (pp. 187–210). Minneapolis: University of Minnesota Press. As Agnew Sees It (1970, May 10) *New York Times*, p. A27.

Asarnow, J.R. & Callan, J.W. (1985). Boys with peer adjustment problems: Social cognitive problems. *Journal of Consulting and Clinical Psychology, 53,* 80–87.

Barron, F.X. (1965). *The psychology of creativity*. New York: Holt, Rinehart & Winston.

Bhatia, K., & Golin, S. (1978). Role of locus of control in frustration-produced aggression. *Journal of Consulting and Clinical Psychology, 46,* 364–365.

Binet, A., & Simon, T. (1973). *The development of intelligence in young children.* New York: Arno Press.

Burks, B.S., Jensen, D.W., & Terman, L.M. (1930). *The promise of youth: Genetic studies of genius* (Vol. 3). Stanford: Stanford Univesity Press.

Camp, B.W. (1977). Verbal mediation in young aggressive boys. *Journal of Abnormal Psychology,* 1977, *86,* 145–153.

Cohen, S., & Oden, S. (1974). An examination of creativity and locus of control in children. *Journal of Genetic Psychology, 124,* 179–185.

Cooke, D. (1985, June 24). Young and gifted: Advantages don't come without cost. *New York Times,* p. A15.

Cowen, E.L., Pederson, A., Babijian, H., Izzo, L.D., & Trost, M.D. (1973). Long-term follow-up of early-detected vulnerable children. *Journal of Consulting and Clinical Psychology, 41,* 438–446.

Coyne, J. (1976). Depression and the response of others. *Journal of Abnormal Psychology, 85,* 186–193.

Dodge, K.A., Schlundt, D.G., Schocken, I., & Delugach, J.D. (1983). Behavioral antecedents of peer social status. *Child Development, 54,* 1400–1416.

Ellis, A. (1975). *A new guide to rational living.* Englewood Cliffs, NJ: Prentice-Hall.

Ellis, H. (1904). *A study of British genius.* London: Hurst & Blackett.

Feffer, M. (1970). Developmental analysis of interpersonal behavior. *Psychological Review, 77,* 197–214.

Feldman, R.D. (1982). *What ever happened to the Quiz Kids?* Chicago: Chicago Review Press.

Flavell, J.H. (1968). *The development of role-taking and communication skills in children.* New York: Wiley.

Fox, L.H., & Washington, J. (1985). Programs for the gifted and talented: Past, present and future. In F.D. Horowitz & M. O'Brien (Eds.), *The gifted and talented: Developmental perspectives* (pp. 197–222). Hyattsville, MD: American Psychological Association.

Galton, F. (1962). *Hereditary genius.* Cleveland: World.

Gardner, H. (1983). *Frames of mind.* New York: Basic Books.

Getzels, J.W., & Jackson, P.W. (1962). *Creativity and intelligence: Explorations with gifted students.* New York: Wiley.

Gilmour, T. (1978). Locus of control as a mediator of adaptive behavior in children and adolescents. *Canadian Psychological Review, 19,* 1–26.

Gould, S.J. (1981). *Mismeasure of man.* New York: W.W. Norton.

Grinder, R.E. (1985). The gifted in our midst: By their divine deeds, neuroses, and mental test scores we have known them. In F. Horowitz & M. O'Brien (Eds.), *The gifted and talented: Developmental perspectives* (pp. 5–36). Hyattsville, MD: American psychological Association.

Gruber, H.E. (1985). Giftedness and moral responsibility: Creative thinking and human survival. In F. Horowitz & M. O'Brien (Eds.), *The gifted and talented: Developmental perspectives* (pp. 301–330) Hyattsville, MD: American Psychological Association.

Guetzkow, H.S. (1968). Differentiation of roles in task-oriented groups. In D.

Cartwright & A. Zander (Eds.), *Group dynamics and theory* (pp. 512–526). New York: Harper & Row.

Heilbrun, A. (1971). Maternal child rearing and creativity in sons. *Journal of Genetic Psychology, 119,* 175–179.

Hollingworth, L.S. (1942). *Children above 180 IQ.* New York: Worth.

Horowitz, F.D. & O'Brien, M. (1985 Eds.) *The gifted and talented: Developmental perspectives.* Washington, DC: American Psychological Association.

Jackson, N.E. & Butterfield, E.C. (1986). A conception of giftedness designed to promote research. In R. Sternberg & J. Davidson (Eds.), *Conceptions of giftedness* (pp. 151–181). Cambridge: Cambridge University Press.

Janos, P.M. (1983). The psychological vulnerabilities of children of very superior intellectual ability. *Dissertation Abstracts International, 44,* 1030A. (University Microfilms No. 83-18, 377)

Janos, P.M., Marwood, K., & Robinson, N.M. (1985). Friendship patterns in highly gifted children. *Roeper Review, 8,* 46–49.

Janos, P.M., & Robinson, N.M. (1985). Psychosocial development in intellectually gifted children. In F. Horowitz & M. O'Brien (Eds.), *The gifted and talented: Developmental perspectives* (pp. 149–196). Hyattsville, MD: American Psychological Association.

Kohlberg, L. (1969). Stage and sequence: The cognitive-developmental approach to socialization. In D.A. Goslin (Ed.), *Handbook of socialization theory and research* (pp. 347–480). Chicago: Rand McNally.

Kohlberg, L., LaCrosse, J., & Ricks, D. (1972). The predictability of adult mental health from child behavior. In B. Wolman (Ed.), *Manual of child psychopathology* (pp. 1217–1284). New York: McGraw-Hill.

Leavitt, H.J. (1951). Some effects of certain communication patterns on group performance. *Journal of Abnormal and Social Psychology, 46,* 38–50.

Lefcourt, H.M. (1982). *Locus of control: Current trends in theory and research.* Hillsdale, NJ: Erlbaum.

Lifton, W.M. (1972). *Groups: Facilitating individual growth and societal change.* New York: Wiley.

Lombroso, C. (1891). *The man of genius.* London: Walter Scott.

Loranger, M. (1984, June). *Social skills in the secondary school.* Paper presented at the Conference on Research Strategies in Children's Social Skills Training, Ottawa, Ontario, Canada.

Manosevitz, M., Fling, S., & Prentice, N. (1977). Imaginary companions in young children: Relationships with intelligence, creativity and waiting ability. *Journal of Child Psychology and Psychiatry and Allied Disciplines, 18,* 73–78.

Meichenbaum, D. (1975). Toward a cognitive theory of self-control. In G. Schwartz & D. Shapiro (Eds.), *Consciousness and self-regulation: Advances in research.* New York: Plenum Press.

Muller, H.J. (1967). *Adlai Stevenson: A study in values.* New York: Harper & Row.

Parker, J., & Asher, S. (1986, April). *Predicting later outcomes from peer rejection: Studies of school drop-out, delinquency and adult psychopathology.* Paper presented at the convention of the American Educational Research Association, San Francisco.

Peterson, L., Mullins, L., & Ridley-Johnson, R. (1985). Childhood depression: Peer reactions to depression and life stress. *Journal of Abnormal Child Psychology, 13,* 597–609.

Piaget, J. (1932). *Le jugement moral chez l'enfant.* Paris: Alcan.

Piaget, J. (1981). *Intelligence and affectivity: Their relationship during child development.* Palo Alto: Annual Reviews.

Putallaz, M. (1983). Predicting children's sociometric status from their behavior. *Child Development, 54,* 1417–1426.

Renzulli, J.S. (1978). What makes giftedness? Reexamining a definition. *Phi Delta Kappan, 60,* 180–184, 261.

Renzulli, J.S. (1986). A three-ring conception of giftedness: A developmental model for creative productivity. In R. Sternberg & J. Davidson (Eds.), *Conceptions of giftedness* (pp. 53–92). Cambridge, England: Cambridge University Press.

Rubin, K.M. (1973). Egocentrism in childhood: A unitary construct? *Child Development, 44,* 102–110.

St. John, R. (1973). *Eban.* London: W.H. Allen.

Sattler, J.M. (1982). *The assessment of children's intelligence and special abilities.* Boston: Allyn & Bacon.

Savage, L. (1985, August). *Empathy in gifted children—gift or curse?* Paper presented at the Sixth world Conference on Gifted and Talented Children, Hamburg.

Schmitz, C.C. & Galbraith, J. (1985). *Managing the social and emotional needs of the gifted.* Minneapolis: Free Spirit.

Spivack, G., & Shure, M.B. (1974). *Social adjustment of young children.* San Francisco: Jossey-Bass.

Sternberg, R.J. & Davidson, J.E. (Eds.). (1986). *Conceptions of giftedness.* Cambridge England: Cambridge University Press.

Stogdill, R. (1948). Personality factors associated with leadership: A survey of the literature. *Journal of Psychology, 25,* 35–71.

Terman, L.M. (1925). *Genetic studies of genius.* Stanford: Stanford University Press.

Terman, L.M., & Oden, M. (1959). *The gifted group at mid-life: Thirty-five years' follow-up of the superior child.* Stanford: Stanford University Press.

Thomson-Roundtree, P., Caldwell, B., & Webb, R. (1981). An examination of the relationship between role-taking and social competence. *Child Study Journal, 11,* 253–264.

Torrance, E.P. (1960). Explorations in creative thinking. *Education, 81,* 216–220.

Van Lieshout, C., Leckie, C., & Van Sonsbeek, B. (1973, July). *The effects of social perspective taking on empathy and role-taking ability of preschool children.* Paper presented to the International Society for the Study of Behavioral Developmnt, Ann Arbor.

Walters, J., & Gardner, H. (1986). The crystallizing experience: Discovering an intellectual gift. In R.J. Sternberg & J.E. Davidson (Eds.), *Conceptions of giftedness* (pp. 306–331). Cambridge: Cambridge University Press.

Weissman, P. (1971). The artist and his objects. *International Journal of Psychoanalysis, 52,* 401–406.

Wolf, T.H. (1973). *Alfred Binet.* Chicago: University of Chicago Press.

Wolfe, T. (1952). The story of a novel. In B. Ghiselin (Ed.), *The creative process* (pp. 186–198) Berkeley: University of California Press.

Yoder, A. (1894). The study of the boyhoods of great men. *Pedagogical Seminary, 2,* 134–156.

2
Peer Acceptance of Gifted Children: The Pedestal Revisited

It is much easier to criticize psychological research than to solve the problems inherent in conducting well-designed studies. Therefore, before reviewing the empirical literature on the peer relations of gifted children, this chapter begins with a summary of the challenges that are inevitably faced by any researcher studying the social behavior of the gifted.

The Challenge of Studying Peer Relations

The importance of studying children's peer relations cannot be disputed. There may be no other aspect of children's behavior that better predicts adult psychological well-being. The connection between childhood social competence and adult mental health has been documented by longitudinal studies conducted in a number of locations. In virtually every case, there is moderate positive correlation between early peer acceptance and whatever measure of adult adjustment is studied (Cowen, Pederson, Babijian, Izzo, & Trost, 1973; Havighurst, Bowman, Liddle, Mathews, & Pierce, 1962; Kupersmidt, 1983; Lambert, 1972; Northway, 1944, Parker & Asher, 1986; Robins, 1966; Rolf & Hasazi, 1977). It is probably the consistency of these findings rather than the size of the correlations that has inspired many new studies as well as intervention programs.

Thus, there is a general consensus that children's social behavior is worth measuring. Unfortunately, there is much less agreement as to exactly *how* it should be measured. The divergent means of measuring social competence derive from varying definitions of this construct (see Dodge, 1985, for fuller discussion). Complicating matters further is the fact that the correlations among different measures of social competence are usually not very large (Gresham, 1981; Hops & Finch, 1982). One of the most fundamental decisions that must be taken by the researcher contemplating the study of the peer relations of gifted youngsters is which measure of social competence to use. The outcome of that decision may substantially determine the results of the study, for reasons explained in the following discussion.

Sociometric Techniques

Most of the longitudinal studies previously cited utilized the children's peers as the primary source of information. There are two major types of sociometric techniques: peer ratings and peer nominations. In a peer rating scale, children are asked to rate their classmates in terms of a given description or series of descriptions. Figure 2.1 is a sample rating scale developed by Asher and his colleagues (Asher, 1985). Respondents are asked to rate their classmates on a 1–5 scale in terms of how much they would like to play (or work) with each child. In a peer nomination

Name _____

EXAMPLES:

How much do you like to play with this person at school?

	I don't like to				I like to a lot
Louise Blue	1	2	3	4	5
Russell Grey	1	2	3	4	5
John Armon	1	2	3	4	5
Andrea Brandt	1	2	3	4	5
Sue Curtis	1	2	3	4	5
Sandra Drexel	1	2	3	4	5
Jeff Ellis	1	2	3	4	5
Bill Fox	1	2	3	4	5
Diane Higgins	1	2	3	4	5
Harry Jones	1	2	3	4	5
Jill Lamb	1	2	3	4	5
Steve Murray	1	2	3	4	5
Jo Anne Norman	1	2	3	4	5
Pam Riley	1	2	3	4	5
Jim Stevens	1	2	3	4	5

HOW MUCH DO YOU LIKE TO PLAY WITH

THIS PERSON AT SCHOOL?	1	2	3	4	5
	I don't like to				I like to a lot

FIGURE 2.1. Sample rating scale sociometric measure.

technique, children would be asked to *name* the classmate or classmates they would most like to play with, work with and so on.

Peers are likely the best judges of a child's peer relations. Sociometric techniques are the best-developed and most valid measure of childhood social behavior. They require little time to administer. However, there are drawbacks. First of all, this method requires access to the peer group. If there is one gifted child in a regular class, one must have the consent of that child's classmates and their parents as well as the participation of the gifted child. Most of the data generated will likely be discarded as not germane to the hypotheses under consideration. This is because only the ratings (or nominations) of the gifted child and of the few others selected for comparison purposes contain any useful information about the peer relations of the gifted.

If one is studying gifted children in special classes or schools, additional questions emerge as to the meaningfulness of sociometric data. Does one obtain information from fellow members of a special class for the gifted? These data may not be without value if those classmates constitute the most meaningful peer group for the gifted children under study. However, the results must not be understood as a portrayal of the acceptance of giftedness among children in general. If one wished to explore the popularity of gifted special class pupils among nongifted peers, one would have to obtain ratings from children with whom the gifted associate during recess or other small portions of the school day. These "part-time" peers may not know the gifted children well enough to meaningfully rate them.

Institutional obstacles may also limit the utility of sociometric techniques. Children generally react positively to them. Hayvren and Hymel (1984) studied children's conversations and interactions after completing sociometric ratings. If there is any change, the children rated become more positive toward each other. However, adults are often more uncomfortable about children's participation in sociometrics than the children are. Asher (1985) discusses some possible solutions to this problem.

Observational Techniques

Children's social behavior has also been studied by means of direct observation. Observers have systematically coded recess play, classroom interaction (especially among preschoolers), and small play groups (LaGreca & Stark, 1986). These methods have undeniable face value: No one can deny that two children interacted if trained, reliable observers witnessed the event. However, it is quite possible that the presence of the observers affected the interaction. Furthermore, some of the most salient aspects of interpersonal relations may not be readily observable, or may be highly infrequent, for example, self-disclosure, aggression, empathy (Furman, 1985). After the first few years of school, academic lessons occupy most of the children's time; there may be little social interaction to observe during these periods (Loranger, 1984). In addition, observational techniques are very expensive and time-consuming. If one were studying the social interaction of gifted and nongifted children, one would likely observe the interaction of peers with one or two children per class. One's team of trained, reliable observers would have to move from place to place; the results might be affected by differences in the physical settings, organization of the different schools, and the like. If one wanted to observe the social behavior of gifted children in special programs, one would face the same limits as with the sociometric procedures. Patterns of interaction among gifted children cannot be interpreted as indicative of the general social interaction of the gifted and nongifted.

Kindergarten teachers have often reported that gifted children tend to isolate themselves in reading corners and avoid "rough and tumble" games. Austin and Draper's (1981) review includes three observational studies of gifted preschoolers. However, these studies did not compare gifted and nongifted classmates in terms of social behavior. In one of the studies, it was found that gifted children who are precocious in reading did in fact isolate themselves somewhat and interact with adults more extensively than gifted nonreaders. An observational study of the social behavior of integrated gifted kindergarteners is planned by the University of Ottawa Children's Social Skills Laboratory in order to establish more conclusively the play patterns of young gifted schoolchildren.

Role-Play Methods

An alternate to direct observation of children's interaction is the use of role play. These instruments are best developed for the measurement of children's assertive behavior but are not necessarily limited to that area. The child is given a situation prompt and demonstrates how he or she would react in that situation. These measures are economical and convenient; very reliable scoring schemes have been developed (Bellack, 1979; Gresham, 1986).

Serious questions have been raised about the validity of role-play techniques. Do they correspond to children's social behavior in real-life situations? It has been remarked that role-play tests may be more reflective of what children *know* than what they *do* (Bellack, Hersen & Turner, 1979). As discussed in the previous chapter, knowing what to do in a social situation is a thinking skill that some have associated with giftedness. However, there is little reason to suspect that the gifted would be any better able to implement this knowledge than any other group. Translating social knowledge to social behavior requires freedom from anxiety and inhibition, as well as reinforcement by others. There has been very little use of role-play tests of social skill with the gifted. Perhaps researchers are wary of finding out what gifted children know but do not do in their relations with peers.

Ratings by Parents and Teachers

Parents and teachers are another important source of information about children's social behavior. Ratings by such significant others enable the researcher to take advantage of the thousands of hours these adults spend with children. Such ratings are easily obtained and economical. Parent and teacher ratings have been well validated as measures of children's attention and self-control (e.g., Conners, 1970). There is some feeling that teachers' ratings have an advantage over those completed by parents because teachers are in a better position to compare a given child with the "norm." Also, they may have less personal investment in the outcome of the assessment.

Although teacher rating instruments have been well developed for many aspects of child behavior, their status as measures of social behavior is unclear. Some studies have found them to be relatively good predictors of other measures of social behavior (see review by Gresham, 1981). Byrne and Schneider (1986) compared teacher ratings of social behavior with pupils' self-ratings. The teachers and pupils rated the children's social behavior using the same items (except for pronouns). The authors found considerable concordance between the teachers' and pupils' ratings on dimensions of self-control, following social rules and conventions, and academic-related social interaction, but little agreement with regard to positive prosocial behavior. In their discussion, Byrne and Schneider speculate that teachers may be best able to rate those social behaviors that directly involve them but not those behaviors that would require them to monitor friendship patterns among children in their classes.

With regard to gifted children, some additional concerns apply. "Halo" effects are a major source of error in all third-party ratings. Teachers sensitive to the scholastic strengths of gifted children may be inclined to rate them as advanced in all areas, including social competence.

Self-Report Scales

The impressions of the children themselves may be the most important source of information about their social behavior. Whether accurate or not, these impressions will, to a considerable extent, determine the psychological impact of peer relations on the individual. This discussion will be continued in Chapter 5. As will be explored in greater detail at that point, one cannot assume that a child's self-report of social behavior corresponds to the social behavior observable to significant others or outside observers. This especially may be the case for the gifted. Let us consider a frequent self-report variable: the number of friends a child has. In contrast with a nongifted child, the ratings of the gifted may reflect a more sophisticated conception of friendship as well as their often-lamented high standards for themselves.

Even if one uses self-report, teacher, or parent ratings, the problem of selecting suitable control groups for the gifted is not fully solved. In some studies, rating scales administered to gifted children are compared with the norms in the manual. While this is not without value, it obscures the fact that social classes, ethnic groups, and neighborhoods have their own norms for social behavior (Achenbach, 1982). There is no way of clearly establishing that the gifted children under study differ from the youngsters in the distant normative group any more than their nongifted peers.

Comparison of Measures

How do these measures of the social behavior of the gifted compare with each other? Table 2.1 displays the results of a reanalysis of the grade 5 and grade 8 data from the study completed by Schneider, Clegg, Byrne, Ledingham, and Crombie (1986). The authors' procedure and results are discussed later in this chapter. As shown, the concordance between different sources of information regarding the social competence of gifted children is rather poor. There are some significant correlations in the table. However, the pattern of findings is not consistent across the two grade levels. Furthermore, the correlations that achieved statistical significance are in every case still very small. These results are not inconsistent with the relations between measures of social competence reported in studies conducted with nongifted children.

A researcher contemplating a study of the social relations of the gifted therefore must be careful in the selection of social competence measures and especially in the interpretation of the findings. If one wishes to make inferences about the peer acceptance of the gifted, one must obtain information from peers of the gifted. The other sources of information are not without value, provided that their interpretation is guided by the true nature of the measure involved. For example, teachers' *impressions* of the peer relations of the gifted are in themselves an interesting phenomenon worthy of study. However, these impressions should not be represented as necessarily indicative of the peers' actual interaction with gifted classmates. Unfortunately, such errors of interpretation abound in textbooks and other writings about the gifted. For these reasons, sociometrics will

TABLE 2.1. Intercorrelations of social competence measures: 54 Grade 5 (above diagonal) and 59 grade 8 (below) integrated, gifted children.

	PN	TR	SR	PR
Peer nominations for social competence (PN)		.23*	.17	.04
Teacher ratings of social participation (TR)	−.14		.26*	.26*
Self-ratings of social self-concept (SR)	.07	−.11		.23*
Parent ratings of social involvement (PR)	.23*	−.14	.31*	

* $p < .05$

constitute the core of the review of the literature that appears later in this chapter, although other measures do provide useful supplements.

The Challenge of Studying the Gifted

The researcher's next hurdle is accurately identifying the gifted subjects and, hopefully, a meaningful comparison group of nongifted peers. Ideally, one would like to select—from a representative, normal population, using reliable, valid measures—children who display exceptional talents—as defined by well-validated criteria—in the areas of intelligence, creativity, task commitment, and others (see discussion of conceptualizations of giftedness in Chapter 1). Of course, this is not scientifically possible at the moment even if one had the time and resources.

"Preselected" Gifted Populations

Many studies are conducted with children in special programs for the gifted and talented. This method has the advantage of permitting the researcher to invest available resources in the study of social competence, not the selection of subjects. When one is interested in the social competence of the gifted, there are some distinct disadvantages. The most devastating of these is the self-selection factor. Even if one can establish that those already in the program are in fact gifted (which would not be too difficult), there is no way of knowing who has been denied admittance to the particular program, or whether any gifted children have not been referred to it because of social relations problems. If gifted children with poor peer relations are overlooked or excluded, one will necessarily overlook the very subjects one most wishes to study. The likelihood of finding that gifted children are socially competent would thus increase. One may also unwittingly "screen out" those gifted children whose parents may have restricted access to special programming. These might include gifted youngsters from culturally diverse backgrounds whose parents may not seek out information about special programs for the gifted and may be uncomfortable in special education proceedings that have become quite legalistic. Using "preselected" subjects also entails using whatever selection criteria are chosen by those in charge of the program. They may not have anticipated a research program when they developed those criteria.

Screening Subjects From a "Normal" Population

One possible means of identifying gifted subjects is to administer a measure or measures of giftedness to an entire population. The first drawback here is cost. One must administer tests to several times more children than will be useful to the study. This alone may entail methodological compromises. One may have to use preexisting measures, such as group tests routinely administered as part of a school testing program. Even if one can introduce measures of one's own selection, economics may dictate the use of group paper-and-pencil measures. As noted by Marland (1972) and Sattler (1982, p. 437), group IQ tests are usually considered inferior to those administered individually in the identification of giftedness. Some gifted children may have learning disabilities, which may interfere with their responses on answer blanks that are to be computer scored. Group and individual IQ tests often yield divergent results. In addition, most group tests yield only a single IQ score and are therefore not useful in identifying youngsters with specific areas of exceptional talent (see discussion of multifactor models of intelligence in Chapter 1).

The challenge of selecting valid measures of giftedness increases when one attempts to go beyond IQ in the identification of gifted subjects. Suppose one wanted to include creativity, for example, in one's screening criteria. Creativity is often defined operationally in terms of divergent thinking. A reliable measure would probably have to specify preset criteria used to determine whether a given response was creative. Thus, a standardized test of creativity may be a contradiction in terms. Cronbach (1984) presented a useful commentary on tests of creative thinking. He noted (p. 262) that their results are unstable and that predictive validity is poor. Different tests of "creativity" also correlate poorly with each other (Cronbach, 1984; Sattler, 1982).

Teacher and parent ratings have also been proposed for the screening of gifted children (e.g., Ciha, Harris, & Hoffman, 1974; Jacobs, 1972; Pegnato & Birch, 1959; Renzulli, Hartman, & Callahan, 1971). As noted by Whitmore (1979, 1980, 1985), these scales often assume positive attitude and motivation. Therefore, there is a distinct danger in using these instruments in a study of social competence. Negative halo effect may well influence the ratings. Because of their negative social behavior, gifted children with peer relations problems may be rated negatively on all attributes and not score in the "gifted range."

Thus, the well-founded move to go beyond IQ in the assessment of childhood giftedness inevitably leads to discussions of babies and bathwater. Nowhere are identification criteria more problematic than in the study of the social relations of the gifted. For reasons explicated in Chapter 1, the results of any such study will depend on the measure used. A study of gifted children identified according to intelligence might well yield conclusions about their social competence that differ dramatically from those of an examination of the peer relations of the highly creative.

How Many Gifted?

Once one has chosen instruments for the identification of gifted subjects, one must then determine a cutoff point for considering subjects as gifted.

Ideally, any such cutoffs should have some empirical support (see the American Psychological Association's *Standards for Psychological and Educational Testing*, 1985). Unfortunately, there are little data that could be useful in determining such cutoffs. However, this decision may have profound impact on results relative to peer relations. As noted in Chapter 1, the social competence of the very highly gifted has often been considered more problematic than that of the "moderately gifted." In some cases, researchers in this area may be in the unusual position of reducing their sample size in order to better test their hypotheses. Any statistics textbook will help calculate the price thus paid.

Volunteer Effect

It is unclear whether the parents of the children in the early studies of giftedness were ever asked to consent to their children's participation. However, ethical standards have by now become very stringent and specific. Schneider et al. (1986) speculate that in the classes under study, consent might not have been received for those gifted children who were experiencing the most severe peer relations problems. The authors were alerted to this possibility by the teacher of one of the special classes for the gifted after he examined the list of pupils for whom consent to participate had been obtained. While the reasons for any such bias is unclear, it is possible that children with social relations difficulties may not wish to rate their shortcomings.

Era Effects

Any contemporary book about gifted children (including the present volume) will document the extended life span of studies of gifted children. It would not be laudable to totally ignore the wisdom of our elders or to erase from memory their perceptive and painstaking research. However, findings must be interpreted in light of the social and intellectual climate of their times. This is particularly applicable to studies of the peer acceptance of gifted children.

A Review of the Empirical Literature

By this point, it is hopefully apparent that any research on the social relations of gifted children is destined to be an adventure in compromise. There are no easy solutions to the methodological problems reviewed. How have researchers responded to these rather weighty challenges? The remainder of this chapter is a critical review of research on the peer relations of gifted children. Primary emphasis is given to studies in which information obtained from peers was utilized. Studies of the social self-concept of the gifted child are reviewed in Chapter 5. Chapter 7 contains a review of research on the effects of special educational programming on the social development of the gifted.

Table 2.2 is a summary of known sociometric studies in which gifted and nongifted children were compared. There is remarkable consistency in the results. Every sociometric study of the peer relations of the gifted child at the elementary school level indicates that they are better accepted than controls!

There are important methodological limitations to many of the studies. The gifted have not always been compared with appropriate controls. For example, Grace and Booth (1958) compared the gifted with their least intelligent classmates, rather than randomly selected peers or a group of average intelligence. In some studies, "gifted" or "superior" was used to refer to children with IQs as low as 120 (e.g., Miller, 1956); based on the distribution of the Stanford-Binet, approximately 14% of the population would thus be considered gifted. However, despite these and other methodological problems, the consistency of the results argues that further replication of these findings may not be a sound investment of research time. Giftedness cannot be seen as a social liability at the elementary school level. Rather, it is usually found to be an advantage.

As indicated, there have been comparably few efforts to extend these findings into the junior and senior high school years. This is understandable, as there are numerous obstacles inherent in the use of sociometric techniques after elementary school. Rotary timetables often make it difficult to identify the student's peer group. For example, if one studies children in a homeroom class in a large community, they may not know

TABLE 2.2. Sociometric studies conducted with high-IQ children.

Author and date	Age range	Results	
Barbe (1954)	Grades 4–7	+	
Heber (1956)	Grades 3–5	+	
Miller (1956)	Grades 4 and 6	+	
Gallagher and Crowder (1957)	Grades 2–5	+	
Grace and Booth (1958)	Grades 1–6	+	
Mann (1957)	Grades 4–6	+	
Martyn (1957)	Grades 4–12	+[a]	NS[b]
Gallagher (1958b)	Grades 2–5	+	
Pielstick (1963)	Grades 4–6	+	
Wood (1965)	Grades 7–8	NS	
Norwood (1977)	Grade 5	+	
Killian (1981)	Junior and senior high school	+	
Schneider et al. (1986)	Grades 5, 8, and 10	+[c]	NS[d]

Note. + = gifted better accepted than controls; NS = no significant differences.
[a] Elementary school.
[b] Junior and senior high school.
[c] Grade 5.
[d] Grades 8 and 10.

each other well enough to meaningfully evaluate their peers. If one studies the acceptance of the gifted pupils in a language or math class, the control group may not be representative, because the gifted are often enrolled in advanced levels of these subject areas.

Despite these difficulties, there are two studies that permit a developmental perspective on the peer relations of the gifted. Martyn (1957) studied the social acceptance of 354 gifted children in elementary, junior high, and senior high schools. The gifted subjects were identified by means of individually administered Wechsler or Stanford-Binet scales (although

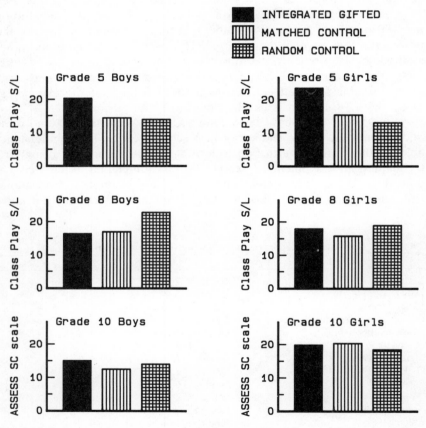

FIGURE 2.2. Peer ratings of social competence: means, all grades. Data from *The Social Consequences of Giftedness in Ontario Schools* by B. Schneider, M. Clegg, B. Byrne, J. Ledingham and G. Crombie, 1986. Unpublished research report, Social Sciences and Humanities Research Council of Canada and Ontario Ministry of Education, SC = Social Competence; S/L = Sociability/Leadership.

for some reason the cutoff scores used, even when converted to standard scores, were not the same for the two measures). Gifted elementary school students were assigned significantly higher acceptance scores than peers. There were no significant differences between the scores of gifted junior and senior high school students and their nongifted peers.

Nearly 30 years later, an identical pattern emerged in a study conducted by Schneider et al. (1986). They collected peer nominations of 204 gifted children in grades 5, 8 and 10. These gifted children were identified on the basis of scores at the 97th percentile or higher on school-administered group IQ tests. There were two control groups. The matched control group consisted of one classmate of each gifted subject matched on the basis of sex, age, and length of enrollment at the school. The random control group consisted of another classmate selected at random. This was done in order to reduce the likelihood of the results being attenuated by differences between the target and control groups on variables not accounted for in the matching procedure. The Revised Class Play procedure (Masten & Morison, 1981) was used for the peer nominations in grades 5 and 8. The ASSESS scales (Prinz, Swan, Liebert, Weintraub, & Neale, 1978) were used in grade 10. The results are depicted in Figure 2.2. The only significant difference, in favor of the gifted group, occurred at the fifth-grade level.

Thus, the consistency of the peer acceptance of the gifted is reduced when a cross-sectional perspective is introduced. Nevertheless, giftedness is not found to be a social liability in the higher grades even though it is no longer an asset. Both studies (Martyn, 1957; Schneider et al., 1986) were conducted in communities that are somewhat atypical: Palo Alto, California, and Ottawa, Ontario, Canada residents far exceed their national averages for education and income. Therefore, the results should be generalized with caution until replicated elsewhere. It would be of particular interest to examine the peer acceptance of gifted children from economically deprived areas. In general, though, it is not inconceivable that many gifted children may have to relinquish the highest levels of social status at puberty.

Instrumentation

Most of the studies reviewed have used peer nomination rather than peer rating scales. As previously discussed, this means that the children were asked to state, for example, which classmate they would most like to play or work with, rather than rating their classmates as in Figure 2.1. These nomination procedures may provide less information than peer ratings on all but "extreme" children (i.e., the asked-for three best-liked students or the two with whom the majority would most like to play). Peer nominations also have been found to be less stable than peer ratings (Asher, Singleton, Tinsley, & Hymel, 1979; Murphy, 1986). However, quite a few of the early studies used the Classroom Social Distance Scale, in which each subject rates every classmate. The findings seem little different from those of the peer nomination studies.

Although few authors question the overall finding that gifted elementary school children are generally well liked by their peers, several of them add case examples that do not follow the general pattern. It is not inconceivable that a minority of gifted children are actively rejected. Unfortunately, the instruments used have rarely been adequate to determine whether this minority is actively disliked ("rejected" in sociometric terms; see Asher, 1985) or simply not included among the three or so "best friends" that the children were required to name in some of the earlier sociometric procedures (e.g., Grace & Booth, 1958; Gallagher, 1958a, 1958b).

Sex Differences

Solano (1976) reported significant differences between pupils' perceptions of hypothetical male and female gifted peers. However, most of the sociometric studies summarized in Table 2.2 were conducted prior to the recent increase in awareness of possible sex differences in studies of children's development. Therefore, very few of the studies included any subsidiary analysis for gender differences in the peer acceptance of the gifted. Killian (1981) found no sex differences between the peers' perceptions of gifted boys and girls, although nongifted girls were regarded more positively than nongifted boys. The identical pattern was found for the peer nominations for social competence in grade 10 only by Schneider et al. (1986). They found no significant sex differences in the peer nominations for social competence in grades 5 and 8.

However, even in these studies, it is possible that sex differences were obscured because the peer nominations were not collected separately by sex (Ledingham, 1981, discusses this procedure). Children of both sexes rated peers of both sexes at the same time. If, in a not implausible situation, boys devalue gifted females, but girls rate them as popular, the effects would cancel each other out and no significant differences would emerge in the analyses. Hopefully, updated sociometric procedures will be employed in future studies to help clarify any sex differences in peer acceptance of the gifted.

Peer Acceptance of the Very Highly Gifted

Since the appearance of Hollingworth's (1942) classic case studies of children with very high IQs (over 180), there has been concern throughout the field for the psychosocial adjustment of this group. There is a widespread feeling that the very highly gifted display less successful peer relations than their moderately gifted counterparts. Some support for this contention can be derived from sociometric studies by Gallagher (1958a) and Gallagher and Crowder (1957). In the study by Schneider et al. (1986), there were significant *negative* correlations within the gifted sample between IQ and peer nomination scores for grades 5 and 8; a nonsignificant trend in the same direction occurred in grade 10. These findings are consistent with several studies of the social and personal adjustment of children with very high IQs in which parent and teacher ratings were used (summarized in Janos & Robinson, 1985). Thus, there is considerable reason to believe that the social status of the very highly gifted is not as consistently elevated as that of the moderately gifted.

Studies Using Rating Scales

As previously detailed, peers are the best source of information about children's peer relations. However, given the many obstacles inherent in the use of sociometric techniques, it is not surprising that many researchers have resorted to the use of rating scales of children's social behavior. The reader is referred to review articles by Austin and Draper (1981) and Janos and Robinson (1985) for more complete surveys of this literature.

Studies in which teacher and parent ratings of gifted children were compared with controls are summarized in Table 2.3. It is obvious from the remarks in the table that these studies have focused on rather divergent aspects of social competence. For that reason, they are not readily comparable.

Nevertheless, it is interesting to note that the social behavior of gifted

TABLE 2.3. Teacher and parent ratings of the social behavior of gifted children.

Author and date	Age range	Results	Remarks on gifted
Gallagher & Crowder (1957) (T)	Grades 2–5	+	Higher in social ability
Nichols (1966) (T)	Adolescents	−	Less sociable than others
Painter (1976) (P and T)	Grade 1	−	Prefer older playmates
Duncan & Dreger (1978) (P)	Grades 11–13	+	Rated as more sociable
Ludwig & Cullinan (1984) (T)	Grades 1–5	+[a]	Have fewer behavior problems
Freeman (1985) (P and T)	?	−	More emotionally troubled
Schneider et al. (1986) (T)	Grades 5 and 8	+	Rated as higher in social participation

Note. P = parent ratings; T = teacher ratings; + = gifted better adjusted than nongifted; − = gifted poorer adjusted than nongifted.
[a] Nonsignificant trend ($p = .06$).

children is not portrayed as positively by adults as by the children's peers. Perhaps adult ratings are colored by presuppositions about the peer acceptance of the gifted. Children may be more tolerant of divergence than we think.

Peer Acceptance of the Creatively Gifted

In the studies previously reviewed, giftedness is defined as high intellect. As expounded in Chapter 1, there are many reasons to believe that highly creative youngsters might not be as well liked as those endowed with precocious academic talent. This possibility was explored by Wallach and Kogan (1965). They found that highly creative young children did display less interest and involvement in social activities than their peers. Nevertheless, they were still well accepted by their peers. IQ mediated this relationship: creative children with high intelligence were high in peer esteem; creative youngsters with lower IQs were not. Again, a developmental perspective on the social status of the creatively gifted is still lacking.

What Differentiates Popular and Unpopular Gifted Children?

Schneider et al. (1986) compared popular and unpopular gifted students in terms of extracurricular activities. There were a total of 204 gifted children in this study, who were attending regular classes, and therefore interacted with nongifted peers on a daily basis. Extracurricular activities were assessed by means of a self-report measure based on the activities and social scales of the Child Behavior Checklist (Achenbach & Edelbrock, 1979). The following item clusters were included: sports, hobbies and games, jobs, organizations, general sociability, and time spent on social life. The results were somewhat inconsistent. At the fifth-grade level, the overall discriminant function did not achieve statistical significance. In grade 8, the 19 gifted children who had achieved the highest peer nomination scores for sociability–leadership (i.e., the highest third) were significantly more involved in school jobs than their gifted counterparts with scores in the lowest third. In Grade 10, two groups were differentiated by involvement in school and community organizations. Thus, peer acceptance of the gifted elementary school child appears independent of involvement in social activities. Outside interests seem to figure more prominently in social acceptance later on. In view of the lack of consistency here, and the potential importance of this information for those involved in counseling the gifted child, further study is clearly needed.

Conclusion

Studies of the peer acceptance of gifted children at the elementary school level have been remarkably consistent in demonstrating that they are well liked. Further attempts to refute this scientific fact may bring few benefits to gifted children. However, the very unanimity of these findings may have discouraged subsequent researchers from putting together the last few pieces of the puzzle. Little is known about peer acceptance of the gifted preschooler. Sociometric studies of the gifted adolescent are quite rare. Early studies of the social status of gifted children have not been updated. As a result, recent advances in sociometric techniques have not been applied in this area. An important example is the lack of data from sociometric procedures administered separately by sex. Almost all studies have identified gifted subjects by means of IQ. The social status of children with specific talents, and of creative children, remains unclear.

Virtually unmentioned in the literature is the possibility that gifted children earn the esteem of their peers by reducing commitment to areas of special talent. Therefore, it is important to consider the childhood peer relations of individuals who have gone on to achieve greatness in various walks of life; that is the focus of the next chapter.

References

Achenbach, T.M. (1982). *Developmental psychopathology*. New York: Wiley.

Achenbach, T.M., & Edelbrock, C. (1979). The child behavior profile II. Boys aged 12–16 and girls 6–11. *Journal of Consulting and Clinical Psychology, 1979, 47,* 223–233.

American Psychological Association. (1985). *Standards for educational and psychological testing*. Washington, DC: Author.

Asher, S.R. (1985). An evolving paradigm in social skill training research with children. In B.H. Schneider, K.M. Rubin, & J.E. Ledingham (Eds.), *Children's peer relations: Issues in assessment and intervention* (pp. 157–171). New York: Springer-Verlag.

Asher, S.R., Singleton, L., Tinsley, B., & Hymel, S. (1979). A reliable sociometric measure for preschool children. *Developmental Psychology, 15,* 443–444.

Austin, A., & Draper, D. (1981). Peer relationships of the academically gifted: A review. *Gifted Child Quarterly, 25,* 129–133.

Barbe, W. (1954). Peer relationships of children of different intellectual levels *School and Society,* 60–62.

Bellack, A.S. (1979). A critical appraisal of strategies for assessing social skills. *Behavioral assessment, 1,* 157–176.

Bellack, A.S., Hersen, M., & Turner, S. (1979). Role play tests for assessing social skills: Are they valid? *Behavior Therapy, 9,* 448–461.

Byrne, B.M., & Schneider, B.H. (1986). Student–teacher concordance on dimensions of student social competence: A multitrait–multimethod analysis. *Journal of Psychopathology and Behavioral Assessment, 8,* 263–279.

Ciha, T., Harris, R., & Hoffman, C. (1974). Parents as identifiers of giftedness: Ignored but accurate. *Gifted Child Quarterly, 18,* 191–195.

Conners, C. (1970). Cortical visual evoked response in children with learning disorders. *Psychophysiology, 7,* 418–428.

Cowen, E., Pederson, A., Babijian, H., Izzo, L., & Trost, M. (1973). Long term follow-up of early-detected vulnerable children. *Journal of Consulting and Clinical Psychology, 41,* 438–446.

Cronbach, L.J. (1984). *Essentials of psychological testing.* New York: Harper & Row.

Dodge, K.A. (1985). Facets of social interaction and the assessment of social competence. In B. Schneider, K. Rubin, & J. Ledingham (Eds.), *Children's peer relations: Issues in assessment and intervention.* (pp. 3–22). New York: Springer-Verlag.

Duncan, J., & Dreger, R. (1978). Behavioral analysis and identification of gifted children. *Journal of Genetic Psychology, 133,* 43–57.

Freeman, J. (1985). Emotional aspects of giftedness. In J. Freeman (Ed.), *The psychology of gifted children.* New York: Wiley.

Furman, W. (1985). What's the point? Issues in the selection of treatment objectives. In B. Schneider, K. Rubin, & J. Ledingham (Eds.), *Children's peer relations: Issues in assessment and intervention* (pp. 41–54). New York: Springer-Verlag.

Gallagher, J. (1958a). Peer acceptance of highly gifted children in elementary school. *Elementary School Journal, 58,* 465–470.

Gallagher, J. (1958b). Social status of children related to intelligence, propinquity, and social perception. *Elementary School Journal, 58,* 225–231.

Gallagher, J., & Crowder, T. (1957). Adjustment of the gifted child in regular classes. *Exceptional Children, 23,* 306–319.

Grace, H., & Booth, N. (1958). Is the gifted child a social isolate? *Peabody Journal of Education, 35,* 195–196.

Gresham, F. (1981). Assessment of children's social skills. *Journal of School Psychology, 19,* 120–133.

Gresham, F. (1986). Conceptual issues in the assessment of social competence in children. In P. Strain, M. Guralnick, & H. Walker (Eds.), *Children's social behavior* (pp. 143–180). New York: Academic Press.

Havighurst, R.J., Bowman, F., Liddle, G., Mathews, C., & Pierce, J. (1962). *Growing up in River City.* New York: Wiley.

Hayvren, M. & Hymel, S. (1984). Ethical issues in sociometric testing: The impact of sociometric measures on interactive behavior. *Developmental Psychology, 20,* 844–849.

Heber, R. (1956). The relation of intelligence and physical maturity to social status of children. *Journal of Educational Psychology, 47,* 158–152.

Hollingworth, L. (1942). *Children above 180 IQ, Stanford-Binet:* New York: World.

Hops, H., & Finch, M. (1982, May). *A skill deficit view of social competence in preschoolers.* Paper presented at the annual meeting of the Association for Behavior Analysis, Milwaukee.

Jacobs, J. (1972). Effectiveness of teacher and parent identification of gifted children as a function of school level. *Psychology in the Schools, 8,* 140–142.

Janos, P.M., & Robinson, N.M. (1985). Psychosocial development in intellectually gifted children. In F.D. Horwitz & M. O'Brian (Eds.), *The gifted and talented: Developmental perspectives* (pp. 149–196). Washington, DC: American Psychological Association.

Killian, J.E. (1981). Personality characteristics and attitudes of intellectually gifted secondary school students. *Dissertation Abstracts International, 42,* 2060A. (University Microfilms No. 81-22, 024)

Kupersmidt, J. (1983, April). *Predicting delinquency and academic problems from childhood peer status.* Paper presented at the meeting of the Society for Research in Child Development, Detroit.

LaGreca, A.M., & Stark, P. (1986). Naturalistic observations of children's social behavior. In P. Strain, M., Guralnick, & H. Walker (Eds.), *Children's social behavior: Development, assessment and modification* (pp. 181–213). Orlando, FL: Academic Press.

Lambert, N. (1972). Intellectual and non-intellectual predictors of high school status. *Journal of Special Education, 6,* 247–259.

Ledingham, J.E. (1981). Developmental patterns of aggressive and withdrawn behavior in childhood: A possible method for identifying preschizophrenics. *Journal of Abnormal Child Psychology, 3,* 353–374.

Loranger, M. (1984, June). *Social skills in the secondary school.* Paper presented to the Conference on Research Strategies in Children's Social Skills Training, Ottawa, Ontario, Canada.

Ludwig, G., & Cullinan, D. (1984). Behavior problems of gifted and nongifted elementary school girls and boys. *Gifted Child Quarterly, 28,* 37–39.

Mann, H. (1957). How real are friendships of gifted and typical children in a program of partial segregation? *Exceptional Children, 23,* 199–206.

Marland, S. (1972). *Education of the gifted and talented.* Washington, DC: United States Government Printing Office.

Martyn, K.A. (1957). *The social acceptance of gifted students. Dissertation Abstracts International, 117,* 2501A–2502A. (University Microfilms No. 23-17, 8).

Masten, A., & Morison, P. (1981, April). *The Minnesota revision of the class play: Psychometric properties of a peer assessment instrument.* Paper presented to the Society for Research in Child Development, Boston.

Miller, R. (1956). Social status and socioempathic differences among mentally superior, mentally typical and mentally retarded children. *Exceptional Children, 23,* 114–119.

Murphy, K.H. (1986). *The sociometric assessment of children's social relations: An examination of the effects of employing nominal versus ordinal scaling.* Unpublished master's thesis, University of Waterloo, Ontario.

Nichols, R. (1966). The origin and development of talent. *Phi Delta Kappan, 48,* 492–496.

Northway, M.L. (1944). Outsiders: A study of the personality patterns of children least acceptable to their agemates. *Sociometry, 7,* 10–25.

Norwood, W.A. (1977). Peer nominations of gifted students: A comparison of students and teachers in recognizing traits of intellectually gifted children. (Doctoral dissertation, University of Southern Mississippi, *Dissertation Abstracts International, 38,* 2346B. (University Microfilms No. 77-22, 885).

Painter, E. (1976). Comparison of achievement and ability in children of high intellectual potential. Unpublished master's thesis, London University. London, England.

Parker, J., & Asher, S. (1986, April). *Predicting long-term outcomes from peer rejection: Studies of dropping out, delinquency, and adult psychopathology.* Paper presented to the American Educational Research Association, San Francisco.

Pegnato, C., & Birch, J. (1959). Locating gifted children in junior high schools: A comparison of models. *Exceptional Children, 25,* 300–304.

Pielstick, N. (1963). Perception of mentally superior children by their classmates. *Perceptual and Motor Skills, 17,* 47–53.

Prinz, G., Swan, G., Liebert, D., Weintraub, S., & Neale, J. (1978). ASSESS: Adjustment scales for sociometric evaluation of secondary-school students. *Journal of Abnormal Child Psychology, 6,* 493–501.

Renzulli, J., Hartmann, R., & Callahan, C. (1971). Teacher identification of superior students. *Exceptional Children, 38,* 211–214, 243–248.

Robins, L.N. (1966). *Deviant children grown-up.* Baltimore: Williams & Wilkins.

Rolf, M., & Hasazi, J. (1977). Identification of preschool children at risk and some guidelines for primary intervention. In G. Albee & J. Joffe (Eds.), *Primary prevention of psychopathology* (pp. 121–152, Vol. 1). Hanover, NH: University Press of New England.

Sattler, J.M. (1982). *Assessment of children's intelligence and special abilities.* Boston: Allyn & Bacon.

Schneider, B.H., Clegg, M.R., Byrne, B.M., Ledingham, J.E., & Crombie, G. (1986). *The social consequences of giftedness in Ontario schools.* Unpublished research report, Social Sciences and Humanities, Research Council of Canada and Ontario Ministry of Education.

Solano, C. (1976, September). *Teacher and pupil stereotypes of gifted boys and girls.* Paper presented at the meeting of the American Psychological Association, Washington, DC.

Wallach, M.A., & Kogan, N. (1965). *Modes of thinking in young children.* New York: Holt, Reinhart & Winston.

Whitmore, J.R. (1979). The etiology of underachievement in highly gifted children. *Journal for the Education of the Gifted, 3,* 38–51.

Whitmore, J.R. (1980). *Giftedness, conflict, and underachievement.* Boston: Allyn & Bacon.

Whitmore, J.R. (1985). New challenges to common identification practices. In J. Freeman (Ed.), *The psychology of gifted children.* New York: Wiley.

Wood, D.W. (1965). An analysis of peer acceptance and perceived problems of gifted junior high school students. *Dissertation Abstracts International, 26,* 4515A. (University Microfilms No. 65-14, 293).

3
Early Peer Relations of the Eminent: A Pilot Exploration

With Helen Bienert

The intensive case study method has a long and hallowed tradition, not only in the study of giftedness, but in the more general exploration of the nature and manifestations of intelligence. Although Binet himself was at times critical of the subjectivity inherent in the case study method, he made extensive use of structured interviews, in particular for his studies of creativity. On many occasions, he emphasized the need for studying the "extremes of population," particularly the intellectually gifted, as a means of best understanding the true nature of intelligence (Wolf, 1973, p. 136).

It is therefore not surprising to find that among the early investigations of "genius" conducted at Stanford University in the 1920s was Cox's (1926) study of the lives of eminent individuals. The 282 cases studied at the time were based on retroactively estimated "IQs." These studies have had a profound impact on the field of giftedness. However, her method of establishing the "fossil IQs" of past geniuses has been described as "a primary curiosity within a literature already studded with absurdity— though Jensen and others still take it seriously" (Gould, 1981, p. 184). The IQ of each of the subjects was estimated by a panel of raters. They would start with an IQ of 100 and add or subtract from there, based on anecdotes provided. Obviously, individuals about whom there is much extant biographical information will be found to be more intelligent (Gould, 1981).

An alternative method for generating a sample of gifted individuals for purposes of intensive case study is to directly classify individuals based on their lifetime accomplishments. Aside from the decided advantages in not using fossil IQs, this method is consistent with the more recent conceptualizations of giftedness discussed in Chapter 1. In contrast with retrospective IQ estimates, it presumably permits inclusion of some aspects of giftedness that are more difficult to study prospectively: motivation, creativity, task commitment. For this reason, the case study approach is advocated by most contemporary theorists who contemplate the definition of giftedness (e.g., Sternberg & Davidson, 1986).

The Goertzels (V. Goertzel & Goertzel, 1962) conducted the best known series of case studies of the eminent who were selected on the basis of accomplishments. Their scrutiny of the biographies and autobiographies of over 400 individuals was updated in 1978 (M. Goertzel, Goertzel, & Goertzel, 1978), when approximately 300 more recent personalities were added to the sample. In their methodology, public interest was the essential indicator of accomplishment. The sample consisted of all individuals for whom at least two biographies were available in a medium-sized public library. This data base has been reanalyzed in a number of ways (e.g., Walberg et al., 1981).

Although the case studies of Cox (1926) and the Goertzels (V. Goertzel & Goertzel, 1962; M. Goertzel et al., 1978), and several smaller scale studies, have focused on the childhood experiences of the eminent, most of the attention is typically devoted to tracing the roots of the individual's talent or genius. Parenting practices were often described in great detail. Although limited, some information about the quality of early peer relations can be gleaned from these studies. For example, McCurdy (1960) examined the biographies of the 20 individuals with the highest IQs in the Cox sample. Among his conclusions was the contention that isolation from other children was often a factor in the emergence of genius. Little detail is presented of the data supporting this view. The Goertzels' texts provide little information as to how the biographies were scanned or analyzed, which statistical treatments were performed (although there are repeated references to statistically significant differences), or the exact significance of the results. Nevertheless, they reported (M. Goertzel et al., 1978, p. 345) that 16% of the eminent were rejected or bullied by peers.

The purpose of the research presented in this chapter was to more systematically describe the childhood peer relations of eminent individuals. In order to best complement other studies of the life histories of individuals who have achieved prominence, we adopted the data bases of both Cox (1926) and the Goertzels (V. Goertzel & Goertzel, 1962; M. Goertzel et al., 1978) as our initial sample. However, no use was made of the retroactive IQ estimates provided by Cox, for the reasons outlined above. Thus, our sample is best defined by the subjects' accomplishments in life. There were several reasons for the selection of this combined sample. First of all, these are the best-known data pools of the type. Both were necessary in order to generate a meaningful sample size, since many cases are typically excluded from the final analyses because of insufficient information about childhood. Finally, the possible biases of the original authors seemed to be complementary. Cox, an associate of Terman, may have been seeking to strengthen the image of the intelligent as invulnerable. On the other hand, the Goertzels, by their case study method, may have paid excessive attention to the more colorful, even pathological aspects of the case histories.

Our initial analysis of the biographies of the individuals we studied was extremely disappointing. Accounts of early childhood peer relations were few. It was, of course, impossible to determine whether this lack of information was attributable to the bias of the biographers, lack of available information, or even to the fact that peer relations were not considered important in the psychological makeup of individuals whose lives were devoted to exceptional contributions in other areas. Understandably, those tracing the early history of the eminent are most interested in uncovering the seeds and roots of that eminence. Furthermore, most of these individuals achieved prominence during adulthood. There may have been little reason to preserve documents attesting to their early friendships or lack of them.

We decided to turn to autobiographies. This ground appeared much firmer, at least on the conceptual level. In retelling one's life experiences, one has undeniable access to information about childhood peer relations. No information might be provided on early friendships, feelings of loneliness or social satisfaction, and the like. Nevertheless, inferences based on this omission are at least based on the choice of the individual under study. There are obvious sources of bias in the autobiography method, however. There is no way of establishing the degree to which the subsample who chose to write their own life histories is representative of the total sample of the eminent personalities. Our pilot study indicated that about one third of the autobiographies of famous people included in the combined Cox–Goertzel (Cox, 1926; V. Goertzel & Goertzel, 1962; M. Goertzel et al., 1978) data base would likely contain useful information about early peer relations. Typically, this information was contained in one of the introductory chapters. Some general descriptor of peer relations was provided, along with anecdotal descriptions of young friends or foes.

Method

Following pilot trials of several rating formats, we adopted a coding system consisting of eight bipolar dimensions:

1. Popular/sociable versus solitary/rejected
2. Outgoing/gregarious versus shy/reserved
3. Happy childhood versus unhappy childhood
4. Leader versus follower
5. Domineering versus submissive
6. Rewarded for brightness or talent versus scorned for brightness or talent
7. Having close, satisfying friendships versus having superficial friendships
8. Having one or more close childhood friends versus having none

It was felt that these dimensions captured both the autobiographers' depictions of the nature of their early peer relations and the psychological impact those peer relations must have had on them. In addition, the distinction was made between overall popularity and having a few close but satisfying friendships—which may be at least as rewarding (Furman &

Robins, 1985). Finally, the impact of early gifted behaviors on social relations was included.

Virtually all autobiographies are organized in chronological order. Our coders scanned all chapters devoted to childhood and did not read or code the rest of the books. Thus, we cannot exclude the possibility that brief references to childhood interspersed with accounts of adult life were overlooked, but we are not aware of any such instances. The coders were explicitly instructed that only the descriptions of early social relations provided by the autobiographers were to be taken into account, not inferences based on other achievements of the individual or accounts of his or her later life. They indicated whether either of the biopolar descriptors characterized the autobiography in question. They could also indicate that the information was unclear or mixed or that there was no information relative to the particular category.

The autobiographies were coded by a trained undergraduate psychology student. Autobiographies of individuals who were not included in the data base were used for training purposes in order to avoid loss of data. During the coding phase, a random sample of 25% of the books were also coded by a psychology graduate student in order to establish interrater reliability. Agreement between the two raters was calculated on the basis of exact agreement for each dimension. Interrater agreement ranged from 73% for

TABLE 3.1. Summary of ratings by area of eminence.

	Area of eminence					
Coding category	Visual arts ($n = 4$)	Literature ($n = 19$)	Performing arts ($n = 9$)	Science ($n = 4$)	Politics ($n = 6$)	Other ($n = 6$)
Popular/sociable	2[a]	6	4	3	5	4
Solitary/rejected	1[a]	9	5	0	1	2
Outgoing/gregarious	2	11	5	3	3	2
Shy/reserved	1	7	4	1	0	4
Happy childhood	2	8	6	1	5	5
Unhappy childhood	2	8	3	1	1	1
Leader	0	5	3	2	2	1
Follower	1	7	3	0	0	2
Domineering	2	8	5	0	2	5
Submissive	0	4	2	0	1	1
Rewarded for talent	2	8	5	1	3	2
Scorned for talent	0	0	2	0	0	0
Close friendships	2	10	6	3	5	1
Superficial friendships	0	6	2	0	0	4

[a] Cell totals do not equal total sample because of missing or uncodeable data.

leader/follower to 100% for some close friendships versus none. The average agreement was 87.2%; rates of agreement exceeded 85% for all dimensions except leader versus follower.

Autobiographies were available for only 72 persons from the Cox (1926) sample, approximately one third of the total. Of these, only 10 contained information about early peer relations. There were a total of 317 entries in the Goertzels (V. Goertzel & Goertzel, 1962; M. Goertzel et al., 1978) sample. Autobiographies with pertinent information were available for 37 of these. Thus, a total of 48 autobiographies were studied in depth. These were clustered in terms of areas of eminence: visual arts ($n = 4$), literature (19), performing arts (9), science (4), politics (6), and other (6). A quantitative summary of the ratings by area of eminence appears in Table 3.1. In view of the small sample, limited statistical analyses was performed on the data. A discussion of these analyses follows a more qualitative summary of the childhood recollections contained in the autobiographies.

Eminence in Visual Arts

Unfortunately, there is often little reason to motivate painters or sculptors to write down their life stories. They have clearly chosen another medium for self-expression.

Grandma Moses (Anna Mary Robertson) described her childhood in the late 19th century as "happy days, free from care or worry" (Moses 1952, p. 4). She spoke of chumships as well as a close relationship with her brother. However, she described herself as "proud in those days" (p. 39), suggesting a touch of childhood arrogance, which seemed not to exact too heavy a toll on her peer relations. Her pleasant childhood contrasted with the sudden thrust of hardship and responsibility that accompanied the onset of her adolescence, when she had to begin supporting herself financially.

Painter Augustus John related details of his childhood with similar fondness. He fraternized openly with the children of other social classes, joining in the pretend "cult of the noble savage" (John, 1975, p. 32). Like the fond childhood memories of Grandma Moses, John's pleasant experiences did not extend into adolescence. He was a moody, somewhat depressed adolescent. One close adolescent friendship compensated for his general aloneness.

Contrasting childhood experiences were reported by sculptor William Zorach. Following immigration to America as a young child, his adjustment to the new culture was very difficult. He wrote of no childhood friendships. His classmates teased him because of his father's foreign ways. Along with other rejected children, he was forced to "run the gauntlet" of physically abusive boys in seventh grade (Zorach, 1967, p. 11). He described himself as disturbed, unhappy, and innocent. His one solace was his woodcarving, which the other children considered quite good. Zorach's contemporary, Alexander Calder, also recalled some physical hazing as a child, but remembers these as somewhat briefer incidents, which he accepted without emotional anguish. His childhood was characterized by many close friendships. He seemed to find friends easily after a change of school. Calder's work was also respected by peers: his workshop was the community "center of attention" (Calder, 1977, p. 21).

Obviously, any inferences made on the basis of only four case studies must be considered very tentative. The psychoanalytic literature portrays an image of the artist's life as one of loneliness and turmoil. Juda (1949) arrived at a somewhat more optimistic conclusion based on her study of 50 prominent German-speaking architects, painters, and sculptors. She found that 39 of these were "psychically normal"; six were diagnosed as "schizoid eccentrics"; only one as a schizophrenic (the remaining four displayed various types of mental deterioration associated with aging). It should be noted that the term *schizoid* implies a withdrawal from social interaction. Juda unfortunately provided no information concerning the onset or duration of the schizoid-eccentric behavior pattern or any childhood forerunners. This study deserves particular attention because the diagnoses were based on personal interviews with the artists not on written records.

In our coding of the autobiographies, we may have stumbled on some clear exceptions that do not adequately represent the childhoods of artists. Perhaps those who experienced the most pain in their childhoods spared themselves the discomfort of writing about it. On the other hand, the writing of an autobiography has been seen as having a cathartic effect for those who have endured heavy emotional strain (Allport, 1942). These limited data are not sufficient to refute the notion that the artist as a child *may* suffer. However, one might look more carefully at any presupposition that the artist *must* suffer. While our sampling methods may be biased in favor of those who had positive life experiences, the psychoanalytic studies are probably not conducted without selection bias as well. Those cases are likely chosen because they illustrate the pathological personality process the author wishes to discuss.

It is particularly encouraging that in all four of the autobiographies studied, the artist's artistic precocity was well recognized during childhood and encouraged by the peer group. Even in the one autobiography that describes negative early peer experience, these are clearly not attributable to the sculptor's talent. Storm clouds of impending adolescent agony seem to hover over the accounts of the artists' preadolescent years. There are simply not enough data here to establish whether this is typical of the lives of artists or merely a reflection of essentially normal adolescent adjustment problems.

Early Peer Relations of Prominent Writers

In contrast with painters and sculptors, eminent writers regularly leave us with written accounts of their experiences. Before discussing their autobiographies, it is again helpful to briefly review previous studies of the psychological adjustment of eminent writers, even though they focus primarily on their adult years. Juda's (1949) sample included 37 eminent German-speaking poets. Of these, only 17 were diagnosed as normal. The rest were found to suffer from the gamut of psychological disorders, ranging from depression to alcoholism to schizophrenia. "Emotional instability" ($n = 4$) was the most frequent single diagnosis. Juda believed that certain neurotic traits, such as instability, hypersensitivity, and depression, might stimulate creative ideas. She considered neurosis, but not psychosis, as beneficial to the poet.

Barron's (1965) conclusions about the psychological adjustment of the 30 creative American writers who participated in his study derive from a methodology that is itself highly creative. He invited the subjects (in groups of 5–10) and members of his research staff to spend a long weekend together in a comfortable, converted fraternity house near the University of California at Berkeley. Although a battery of psychological tests were administered, the emphasis was on the participants' getting to know each other through casual if intensive contact; "a wine cellar and fireplace added to the amenities." At the end of the weekend, the staff members rated each of their "guests." The writers were described as independent, "esthetically reactive," and intellectual. The staff members considered them interesting as persons, but not necessarily sociable or socially at ease. Their MMPI profiles indicated higher pathology than the average for the population at large. The average creative writer scored in the upper 15 percent on all scales of psychopathology included in the study. However, Barron's data also indicate that the writers were high on ego strength and resourcefulness in solving problems. Thus, they may experience more problems but would likely be better at overcoming them. Of course, the generality of Barron's findings is no greater than the representativeness of the sample. Perhaps the least sociable and poorest adjusted of writers might not wish to join a live-in weekend assessment. Others may have simply been reticent to spare the time.

Andreasen and Canter (1975) were motivated by the suicides of several famous writers, especially Sylvia Plath, Anne Sexton, John Berryman, and Randall Jarrell, to conduct a case study of 15 writers who participated in the University of Iowa writing workshop. These were compared with a control group of 15 individuals in professions outside the creative arts who were matched for age and education. Interviews revealed that nine of the writers had seen psychiatrists, eight were treated with psychotropic drugs, and four had been in psychiatric hospitals. Six met the criteria for secondary diagnosis of alcoholism. Statistically significant differences were found between the writers and controls on all indices of psychopathology. Andreasen and Canter speculated that a lonely, sensitive, and rejected childhood may have been among the etiological factors (1970, p. 197).

How well do the childhoods of the writers in our present sample bear out these speculations? Fortunately, 19 autobiographies containing descriptions of early peer relations were available for individuals included in the combined Cox–Goertzel data pool. Indeed, these data were not without instances of childhood loneliness, solitude, and rejection. These painful early experiences will be summarized in chronological order.

Edward Gibbon (1966) described his childhood as not being without its happy hours (p. 18). Nevertheless, he characterized himself as timid and reserved (p. 33). Although he was "reviled and buffeted" by his youthful peers, this was attributed to "the sins of my Tory ancestors" (p. 33). His punishment for misbehavior was being sent to a room to be on his own for several hours. He remembers actually enjoying this experience, because it enabled him to escape the dreaded "exercises of the school and the society of my equals" (p. 41). Gibbon found solace in his reading and in the friendship of one intimate acquaintance.

Dramatist Count Vittorio Alfieri (1862) described a childhood characterized by "a solititude in which I found my Master, but which also subjected me to melancholy" (p. 23, translated from the French). As a child he was prone to extremes of behavior, ranging from excessive timidity to forceful obstinacy (p. 27). Both of these extremes have been associated in modern psychological literature with peer rejection. It is therefore not surprising that he became the "constant toy" of his peers, who called him a "swine" (p. 17). These taunts led to deep feelings of depression.

A century later, novelist Phyllis Bentley described herself as a tomboy prone to outbursts of temper. At the same time, she was "perfect bullying material: physically weak, mentally precocious, emotional, too easily reduced to tears. . . . The others whispered together, glancing derisively at me from time to time" (Bentley, 1962, p. 48). This picture improved somewhat when she was transfered to a school in an Ursuline convent. Her contemporary, Enid Bagnold, was a "big, boastful, unwarned child" (Bagnold, 1970, p. 23), who was generally lonely and teased because of her chubbiness. Novelist Catherine Cookson (1971) spent her childhood fighting against the perceived pity of her peers. Her internal tension was manifest in frequent fights; she alternately assumed the role of bully and victim.

Playwright Emlyn Williams went through the motions of playing games with other children, although he never thought of them as people he might like to talk to (1961, p. 31). His comrades enjoyed his clowning more than he did; they were as entertained as he was embarrassed. Although not openly rejected, Williams invested little emotion in childhood peer relations. Companionship did not help him master his inner feeling that something was missing (p. 31).

Novelist Sean O'Faolain reported that throughout his childhood he did not have a single friend (1967, p. 53). This may have been the result of strict parents denying him permission to participate in most of the activities valued by his peers. Eventually, he learned to "love loneliness" (p. 57). Similar reverence for being alone was reported by Victor Pritchett (1968, p. 91). He described himself as an offensive "prig" who envied the success of "boys who lived for the minute and for the latest craze" (p. 109). He longed to join the "small secret society of jocks" (p. 122), but was systematically shut out until he handed in his first story as an adolescent. Thereafter, his writing enhanced his reputation; he remembers one boy interrupting his push-ups to send a flattering joke his way (p. 155). Similarly, William Thackeray found that childhood was "a very lonely business" (1978, p. 7), until his talent at figure drawing put him "cosily in the middle of a circle of friends."

Writers With Positive Early Peer Relations

The preceding essentially negative experiences in childhood peer relations are counterbalanced in our sample by a substantial number of writers who were quite well accepted by their young comrades. Goethe (1848, p. 36) found quite early that he could easily surround himself with reverent companions by telling stories. However, he seems to have developed a special circle of close friends, of which he was something of a leader. He mentions the disdain of other children (p. 49), against which he and his associates defended themselves quite aggressively. In terms of sociometric theory, Goethe would probably be best classified as "controversial."

Harriet Martineau seems to have derived satisfaction from a single very close companion, although in general her childhood was quite unhappy, to the extent that she contemplated suicide (Martineau, 1969, p. 18). While she reports hating herself every day (p. 41), these feelings are attributed to her deafness and ill health. Solace came from religion, intellectual life, and the company of a friend she met at age seven.

George Sand is most eloquent in describing the importance of her early associates. Although she enjoyed these friendships thoroughly, she was aware that, if she allowed herself to pursue social life too much, her creative life would suffer. "...I was weary of idleness, of yielding to the caprices of my companions or following their lead, tired, in short, of our long-continued, systematic rebellion against discipline" (1978, p. 122). This conversion to self-commitment eventually led Sand to a state of "constant ecstasy" brought about by becoming "orderly, obedient and industrious" (1978, p. 146).

Hugh Miller also achieved satisfaction from early perseverance at his writing (1889, p. 47). Support for his commitment was buttressed by a young school chum who "believed in me" (p. 77). His stories earned him the esteem of his classmates (p. 88). While he did not take part in the usual childhood games and activities, he was by self-description a leader, sometimes attracting a following of 10–12 school fellows, on whom he was a "potent influence" (p. 140).

Herman Hesse described himself as an active, happy boy. He remembers having no trouble "playing the role of ringleader or of the admired one or the man of mystery. For years at a time I kept my younger friends and relations respectfully convinced of my literally magic power" (1972, p. 5). However, in adolescence, his rebellious, difficult nature cost him his social success.

Although he was the sensitive "baby" of the family, John Lehmann managed to form a number of friendships that he cherished. These helped compensate for the lack of a brother, which he always wanted. He regretted leaving his friends and happy childhood to go off to Eton at age 14. Once there, he nonetheless developed a new network of friends and became popular by becoming the school storyteller (Lehmann, 1969).

Novelist R.K. Narayan managed to find a circle of friends, even though he was the only Brahmin boy in a predominantly Christian school. This may have been facilitated by being gregarious and something of a follower by disposition (Narayan, 1974). In contrast, Evelyn Waugh achieved social success by acting as a mischievous, assertive leader. When teased by a larger fellow on a single, exceptional occasion, he responded to the challenge by winning a public wrestling–boxing match from which both contestants would surely have been disqualified had a referee been present (Waugh, 1976).

Playwright Tennessee Williams started school as a "little boy with a robust, aggressive, almost bullying nature" (1975, p. 11). Although his mother did not approve of his potential comrades, he seemed quite popular, despite his having moved into a new neighborhood and his isolation during a bout of diphtheria. He would often join other children, "joyfully" (p. 14), in neighborhood pranks. This happy childhood gave way to an adolescence in which his "problems took their most violent form in a shyness of a pathological degree" (p. 17).

Thus, a wide variety of early peer backgrounds characterized the writers in our sample. About half the recollections of early social relations displayed omens of the psychosocial maladjustment that has often been found in studies of adult writers. No stereotype of the writer as a child seems appropriate. They were bullies and bullied, quiet and loud, serious and jovial, happy and miserable. But there is one important common thread—in virtually every case, the precocious creative talent was a source of satisfaction and acceptance.

Performing Artists

The nature of the performing arts dictates demands on the artist in terms of social relations that are very different from those placed on painters, sculptors, composers, or writers. Their training and development require no less task commitment than other artistic endeavors. However, actors cannot productively pursue their craft in isolation. The social skills required to help bring about one's "fortuitous" discovery, and thereby the chance to earn a living at one's chosen occupation, have been documented in films since the 1930s. The "audience factor" applies, to a lesser extent, to such performing arts as orchestral music and dance.

There is considerable market demand for biographies and autobiographies of performing artists. Our sample included nine performing artists, all from the Goertzels' data pool.

Edward G. Robinson (1973) recovered quickly from his early move to New York. Although among the "contingent that complained in class" (p. 27), he was nominated to be class president. His impression was that his outward composure masked his inner insecurity; the disguise was highly effective. His acting talent was recognized early and put to use by teachers. He recalls being put in charge of rehearsals for school plays.

Pianist Arthur Rubinstein's childhood was marred by sharp discord with his family. A "born extrovert" (1973, p. 34), he resented being held back from playing with other children and rejoiced when he was finally allowed to do so. His piano playing was greatly admired by his contemporaries. Most of his friendships were with other creative children; these relationships appear to have been intense and satisfying.

The shy young Helen Hayes, in contrast, was known as "the little white mouse" (1968, p. 15). She had no friends and did not miss having any. She remembers her shyness as having affected her early acting ability. Totally absorbed in her acting, she had no desire to join the offstage group games of the children who had bit parts at the theater. As a "principal," no one expected her to associate with them. Actress (and, later, writer) Maya Angelou (1969) was also not included in other children's games. However, she was profoundly and miserably lonely.

Ethel Waters felt that she never was a child (1951, p. 1). She was a crafty young leader of a street gang, sometimes sneered at, but very capable of holding her own. She began her singing career at age 5; even then she was called back for encores. She remembers wanting to be liked but putting no effort forth to establish friendships. She would wait until "they discovered my remarkable qualities" (p. 30). This would usually suffice. Most other children were her eager friends; she would help them out by providing precise definitions of profane expressions they had heard.

Dancer Margot Fonteyn spent much of her childhood in a world of grown-ups. She was shy, timid, and very critical of herself, although not without a certain rebellious streak (Fonteyn, 1975). She remembers not having been attracted to most other children but did manage to strike up a few close friendships, especially with other girls who were physically small. Nevertheless, she experienced profound feelings of inferiority throughout childhood and always felt like an outsider.

Peter Ustinov (1977) overcame his introverted inclinations to become a "social animal" (p. 38), quite popular with the other boys in his school. He was teased, but not maliciously, because of the German sound of his original name and because of his weight. He earned respect by becoming the local expert on automobiles. He had many "buddies," but these relationships were not particularly intense, "...I do not believe friends are necessarily the people you like best, they are merely the people who got there first" (p. 68).

Marilyn Monroe's (1974) unhappiness and loneliness began in childhood. She was called dumb and teased because of her orphan's clothes. Adolescence brought more acquaintances, but not more friends. She became the object of both scorn and admiration, when she borrowed her sister's makeup and tight sweater.

These case examples illustrate the diversity of child peer relations among those who have achieved fame in the performing arts. Their choice of career, and success at it, may reflect, in part, a compensation for earlier loneliness and rejection or an extension of childhood leadership qualities.

Scientists

The best-known studies of the personal traits of accomplished scientists were conducted by Anne Roe. Her study of 22 eminent physicists and chemists (Roe, 1951a) utilized intensive personal interviews as the major source of information. Of the 114 pages of the monograph, only four are devoted to psychosocial adjustment. Unfortunately, a developmental perspective is not really provided. As in other studies of this type, most of the attention is devoted to early family history, intellectual stimulation, and career choice. Nevertheless, Roe concluded that the subjects' social development was slow and that throughout life they displayed little interest in social relations. Mitroff arrived at a similar conclusion in his study of scientists involved with the Apollo space program (Mitroff, 1974).

Even less information about childhood is contained in Roe's (1951b) study of 20 well-established biologists. In that study, projective tests of personality were the most salient measure. Roe found that, despite their superior intellectual ability, the Rorschach inkblot records of the biologists contained fewer than average images of human beings engaged in interpersonal activity. Consistent with Rorschach literature to this day, this was interpreted as a further indication of the scientists' lack of sensitivity to, and interest in, human relations. The validity of Rorschach responses as measures of personality has been hotly debated and is obviously outside the scope of this volume.

Unfortunately, our sample contained only four scientists, all from the Goertzels sample. This included anthropologist Margaret Mead, who should not really be compared with the physical and biological scientists studied by Roe. Therefore, inferences from our data are made with considerable caution. We shall consider these cases in the context of the "rule" proposed by Roe (1951a; 1951b) that scientists have little interest in interpersonal relationships and that this lack of interest is evident from childhood.

Benjamin Franklin was a leader among the boys and not always a positive influence on the group. Although frequently chided for his "singularity" (1950, p. 20), he remembered always being allowed to govern the group of boys when they went out in boats or canoes. Nevertheless, he most valued his intimate friendship with another "bookish lad in the town" (p. 18).

Charles Darwin as a boy had many friends (1972, pp. 29–31), though he also remembered enjoying long, solitary walks ("what I thought about I know not," p. 29). Although he described his disposition as affectionate (p. 31), he was, like Franklin, not always a positive influence. In particular, he enjoyed making up false stories in order to generate excitement (p. 27). His intellect was well admired. One of his respected tricks was his use of a collection of old verses, which with the help of friends, would be rewritten to pertain to any subject (p. 29). Because of his work in chemistry, he was nicknamed "Gas" by his classmates; it is not clear whether this nickname was affectionate or scornful. The headmaster definitely did not approve of his scientific bent.

Biologist Julian Huxley (1970) provided fewer recollections of peer success. He remembered being applauded by the group for his performance in a class play (p. 32). He considered himself a vain and temperamental child. Although he enjoyed participating in cricket and other sports, there are some recollections of peer rejection. As an adolescent at Eton, he was told that he was no longer wanted by two or three chums whose company he valued; he was shattered as a result.

Simply stated, these three case studies do not support Roe's (1951a; 1951b) contention that scientists have little interest in human relations. Even Huxley's negative experience had a profound emotional impact on him. Again, we may have stumbled upon exceptions to the rule. Perhaps those scientists with the most human interest take the time to share their life histories with future generations.

Margaret Mead (1972) was very much in the center of the social group as a child. She remembered organizing all sorts of games, plays, and performances. She was the protector of little girls; she would read and summarize books for them. She developed a close, "non-sentimental" friendship with the male co-leader of the 16-member core group in the neighborhood, "the first of many friendships based on collaboration" (p. 73).

Statesmen

The ability to achieve eminence in politics and world affairs requires a special type of social skill. These individuals must be able to readily form pleasing relationships with a wide variety of people and maintain a public image of sociability and trust. These relationships do not have to be of any great depth. Thus, the social skills involved may not necessarily correspond with those needed to establish more enduring friendships. In any event, the Goertzels (M. Goertzel et al., 1978, p. 223) concluded that political personalities are seldom rejected by childhood peers.

Indeed, four of the five eminent statesmen studied here were popular as children. Unfortunately, the fifth, Conservative M.P. Sir Oswald Mosly, offered no reasons (or evidence) for his provocative statement that "few things are more overrated than the effect of childhood experiences on later life" (1968; p. 7), and he provided little description of his childhood peer relations.

Henry Cabot Lodge (1975) thoughout life maintained many intimate friendships that started in childhood. He related having many satisfying peer experiences throughout his childhood. What he described as his early "cautiousness" (p. 71) may in fact be early signs of the ability to be tactful and "diplomatic." His penchant for youthful mischief may be the "common touch" that politicians are said to require. Nevertheless, he was referred to at times as a "miserable little dig" because of his high marks in school.

Although Golda Meir's (1976) childhood was not a consistently happy one, she was an organizer of other children from age 11, when she orchestrated a fundraising event for school textbooks. She made friends easily and, like Cabot Lodge, maintained lifelong contact with childhood companions. Soviet general Marshal Zhukov (1971) also reported many close childhood friendships despite the fact that he was poor, hungry, and overworked as a youngster.

Hubert Humphrey's father encouraged his son to get to know everybody (Humphrey, 1976), including children from the "wrong side" of the tracks. Young Hubert shared his classmates' interests in team sports and drama. He was convinced since his school years that "my generation, particularly I, could make things right with the rest of the world".

Although our sample of politicians is small, these recollections are consistent with the Goertzels' finding that political leaders are rarely rejected as children. Despite the superficial likability that may be required in politics, the childhood friendships they reported seem to be among the longest enduring, most satisfying, and least superficial in our sample.

Other Areas of Eminence

Philosopher John Stuart Mill was kept away from other children in order to pursue the intensive educational regimen imposed by his father (Mill, 1963). Although this did not prevent him from having a happy childhood, he grew up to be "disputatious," and he regretted his father's failure to correct this. He defended himself well in verbal debates with older boys.

Jean-Paul Sartre, similarly, had a very solitary childhood, although he did not characterize it as thoroughly miserable (Sartre, 1981).

Newspaper magnate Lord Beaverbrook was one of the "bad boys in the town" (p. 35). Although "naughty" (p. 28) and "audacious," he succeeded in forming a number of close childhood friendships (Beaverbrook, 1965). Publisher Leonard Woolf was shy and introspective, but subject to outbursts of temper (Woolf, 1970). His early peer relations are probably best described as mixed.

Headmaster A. S. Neill of Summerhill School was a clumsy child, a "coward" (1972, p. 42) prone to hero worship. He would tutor more physically adept classmates in exchange for them beating up children who attacked him. Despite his general unpopularity, he did manage to initiate some satisfying peer relationships.

Quantitative Analysis

Statistical analysis was limited to the most salient dimension, popular/sociable versus solitary/rejected. Most of the cell frequencies in Table 3.1, in which the case studies were classified by area of eminence, were too small for statistical treatment. Therefore, larger groupings were formed according to several dimensions of interest. The results are depicted in Figure 3.1.

CREATIVE ARTS

A group of 24 creative artists was formed by combining the codings of visual artists, writers, and musicians. These were contrasted with a comparison group ($n = 13$) comprised of scientists, political and business leaders, and educators. As indicated in Figure 3.1, a disproportion of creative artists were solitary or rejected as children. Chi-square analysis indicated that this difference in proportions approached statistical significance ($p = .10$).

GENDER DIFFERENCES

A greater proportion of eminent females were coded as having childhood peer relations characterized by rejection or loneliness. This difference in proportions also approached statistical significance.

ERA AND BIRTHPLACE EFFECTS

The early peer relations of eminent persons born in Europe were somewhat less successful than those of counterparts born in North America. In addition, those born before 1900 tended to fare better with their childhood

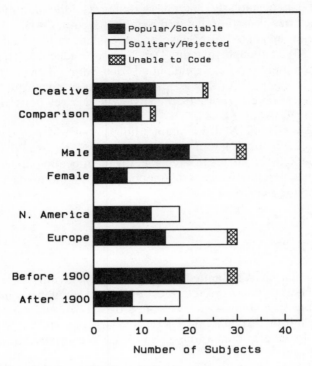

FIGURE 3.1. Results of quantitative scoring by major category.

peers than those born afterward. Neither of these trends was statistically significant.

DOMINEERING CHARACTERISTICS

One final aspect of the quantitative scoring is worthy of attention. As indicated in Table 3.1, a very large proportion of the eminent were rated as having been domineering or bossy during childhood. This negative trait surely exacted a toll on their social acceptance. However, these "pushy" qualities may have been of some advantage in helping them achieve public recognition.

Conclusions

Let us begin with the most encouraging conclusion. Aside from the classmates' jealous scorn of adolescent Marilyn Monroe's tight sweater and the peers' aloof neutrality toward young Helen Hayes' thespian precocity, there are no indications of childhood peers punishing or rejecting the young eminent because of their emerging talents or gifts. Rather, the peers seemed to admire and reinforce the special contributions of most of the children studied. Even those not specifically rewarded for their early accomplishments seemed to regard their special areas of talent as sources of solace and pride. Those who were rejected seem to have been so treated for reasons that often incur rejection for nongifted children as well: unattractive physical appearance, aggressiveness or social withdrawal, ethnic or racial differences.

The degree of rejection in this sample is certainly higher than in the population at large. To some degree, this must be an artifact of our methodology, because the autobiographical method leads to overrepresentation of writers, who appear to experience childhood rejection to a higher degree than those of other areas of excellence. Therefore, we have no reason to dispute the Goertzels' unexplained conclusion that 16% of the eminent in their sample had experienced childhood rejection (M. Goertzel et al., 1978). While we must again refute the hypothesis that the majority of gifted children are disliked as youngsters, the future eminent do not, as a group, seem as well liked as the subjects in the empirical studies summarized in Chapter 2. Perhaps one of the distinctions discussed in Chapter 2 applied here: The very highly gifted may be less respected than those who are moderately gifted.

These data clearly support previous findings that artists and writers experience early peer rejection and unhappy childhoods to a greater extent than other gifted children. Nevertheless, suffering does not appear to be a necessary condition for the emergence of creativity. The number of creative artists with successful childhood peer relations seems essentially comparable to the number with unsuccessful relations. For those who achieved peer acceptance, the challenge must surely have been to maintain commitment to their own areas of excellence in spite of the tempting diversions of childhood social life.

"Egghead" stereotypes apply only to a minority of the young eminent-to-be. Some were indeed bullied, but, contrary to popular impression, a fair number were bullies themselves. In some cases (e.g., Catherine Cookson, 1971), the determination to fight peers seems similar in tone to the determination to excel.

Limits of This Methodology

The study of autobiographical documents has a long tradition in psychology. Many contemporary psychologists eschew this type of research because of its inherent subjectivity. However, there have been a number of recent appeals for the resurrection of the personal narrative as a psychological research tool (e.g., Taylor, Robinson, & McCormick, 1986) because of its ability to capture the complexity and vividness of personality dynamics. Fortunately, enthusiasm for this method has been appropriately tempered by awareness of its inherent limitations. These were best summarized by Gordon Allport (Allport, 1942), a keen advocate of this type of inquiry. The following presentation of the limits of the methodology described in this chapter will parallel Allport's summary of the criticisms leveled against the use of personal documents in psychology.

Unrepresentativeness of Sample

Allport (1942) noted that only a minority of individuals create written records of their mental processes or personalities. He cited Murphy, Murphy, and Newcomb's (1937) observation that these are frustrated individuals with a need to "talk out" their problems. As mentioned above, we believe that it is also possible that a famous person who has achieved acceptance and fame may wish to keep painful past memories well buried. Even though we cannot establish the direction of the sampling bias, we cannot assume that autobiographies constitute an adequate sample of the populations specified. The conclusions presented above are limited by our small sample size. Nevertheless, a larger sample of autobiographies would still not be necessarily representative of the population.

Furthermore, the eminent, whether or not they have left us with autobiographies, may not be truly representative of the gifted. The Goertzels (M. Goertzel, et al. 1978) pointed out that eminence is determined not only by the quality of an individual's achievements but by society's attributions about these achievements. The scientist who one day discovers a cure for cancer may be little different in terms of early personality and peer relations from colleagues who fail to achieve that breakthrough. The only difference between them may be the accident of stumbling upon the guilty organism. However, in other instances there may be a specific social skill that helps individuals propel themselves to eminence.

Nonobjectivity and Unverifiable Validity

Personal documents are by nature subjective. Individuals' accounts of their lives may not correspond with objective reality. Allport provided two replies. The first is that "extreme objectivism has disclosed its own weakness. The resurgence of phenomenology has brought back to favor the personal report" (1942, p. 127). The second is that the personal document ideally should not be considered in isolation but together with other information about the individual. Unfortunately, this cross-validation is not possible in the case of the early peer relations of the eminent. There is little other information available about the early peer relations of these individuals. We might speculate that if the peers of the eminent had written their own autobiographies, their descriptions of relations with the eminent might reflect a different tint, although that shade might be darker or lighter than those previously reviewed.

Motivational Considerations

Critics of the personal document method have pointed out that individuals are often not aware of unconscious drives and motives. The repression of personal shortcomings is not an uncommon defense mechanism; deficits in social skills may thus be downplayed. On the conscious level, individuals may have reasons to manipulate psychological portraits of their childhoods. Conversely, some may experience a need to enhance their identification with suffering artists by retroactive embellishment of their own suffering. Allport pointed out that the motives in deception are often complex:

> ...Perverse exhibitionism is not uncommon. The implicit reasoning seems to be, "Am I not wonderful because I see so many defects and blemishes in my character?" To find oneself so altogether blameworthy is as suspicious as to find oneself altogether blameless. Furthermore, in self-excoriating statements it is often true that some secrets are deliberately hidden. (1942, p. 139)

If such complexity and creativity apply to the motivation behind all personal documents, we cannot be confident that the life stories of the creatively eminent are fully bereft of such distortions. In addition, the eminent may have opinions as to how childhood giftedness is best nurtured. Their own childhood memories may have been modified to support these opinions.

Errors of Memory

One's memory of events that took place in childhood may be clouded by forgetfulness, selective recall, or unconscious influences. The autobiography of one member of our sample, eminent publisher Leonard Woolf, contained the following comments on the validity of memoirs:

> ...I wish I could recall vividly what it felt like to be a boy of twelve or thirteen... (p. 68). Some of the things which one seems to remember from far, far back in infancy are not, I think, really remembered; they are family tales told so often that eventually one has the illusion of remembering them....What genuine glimpses one does get...seem to show that the main outlines of one's character are molded in infancy and do not change. (1970, p. 22)

Alfred Adler (Ansbacher & Ansbacher, 1956) maintained that the distortions in one's early childhood recollections fundamentally reflect an individual's cognitive style and personality. Therefore, early childhood recollections are studied extensively in Adlerian personality assessment. Challenging Freud's views regarding the impact of early life events, Adler believed that it is the person's subjective experience of the events, not objective reality, that determines their psychological importance.

Suggestion for Future Exploration

It is unlikely that a much larger sample of autobiographies of the eminent with useful information about early peer relations is available. Furthermore, the limits of this method previously discussed would not be fully remedied by a larger sample size. Perhaps we would learn more about society's nurturance of giftedness by diverting some attention to the personal narratives of individuals who seem as children to have the potential for gifted behaviors but who do not display these behaviors as adults.

References

Alfieri, V. (1862) *Mémoires de Victor Alfieri (Bibliotheque des mémoires)*. Paris: Firmin Didot Frères, Fils et Cie.

Allport, G.W. (1942). *The use of personal documents in psychological science*. New York: Social Science Research Council.

Andreasen, N., & Canter, A. (1975). Genius and insanity revisited. In R. Wirt, G. Winokur, & M. Roff (Eds.), *Life history research in psychopathology* (pp. 187–210). Minneapolis: University of Minnesota Press.

Angelou, M. (1969). *I know why the caged bird sings*. New York: Random House.

Ansbacher, H.L., & Ansbacher, R.R. (Eds; 1956). *The individual psychology of Alfred Adler*. New York: Harper Row.

Bagnold, E. (1970). *Enid Bagnold's autobiography*. London: Heinemann.

Barron F. (1965). *The psychology of creativity*. New York: Holt, Rinehart & Winston.

Beaverbrook, W.M. (1965). *My early life*. Fredericton, New Brunswick, Canada: Beaver Press.

Bentley, P. (1962). *O dreams, o destinations*. London, England: Victor Gallancz.

Calder, A. (1977). *Calder*. New York: Pantheon.

Cookson, C. (1971). *Our Kate*. Indianapolis: Bobbs-Merrill.

Cox, C. (1926). *Genetic studies of genius: The early mental traits of three hundred geniuses* (Vol. 2). Stanford: Stanford University Press.

Darwin, F. (Ed.). (1972). *The life and letters of Charles Darwin*. (Francis Darwin, Ed.) New York: AMS Press.

Fonteyn, M. (1975). *Margot Fonteyn: Autobiography*. London: Howard & Wyndham, Ltd.

Franklin, B. (1950). *The autobiography of Benjamin Franklin*. New York: Random House.

Furman, W., & Robins, P. (1985). What's the point? Issues in the selection of treatment objectives. In B. Schneider, K. Rubin, & J. Ledingham (Eds.), *Peer relations in childhood: Issues in assessment and intervention* (pp. 41–56). New York: Springer-Verlag.

Gibbon, E. (1966). *Memoirs of my life*. London, England: T. Nelson & Sons.

Goertzel, M., Goertzel, V., & Goertzel, T. (1978). *300 Eminent personalities*. San Francisco: Jossey-Bass.

Goertzel, V., & Goertzel, M. (1962). *Cradles of eminence*. Boston: Little, Brown.

Goethe, J. (1969). *The autobiography of Johann Wolfgang Goethe: Truth and poetry from my own life* (J. Oxenford, Trans.). London: Henry G. Bohn. (Original work published 1893)

Gould, S. (1981). *The mismeasure of man.* New York: W.W. Norton.

Hayes, H. (1968). *On reflection: An autobiography.* New York: M. Evans.

Hesse H. (1972) *Autobiographical writings.* (T. Ziolkowski, Ed; D. Lindley, trans.), New York: Farrar, Straus & Giroux (original work published 1945).

Humphrey, H. (1976). *The education of a public man: My life and politics.* New York: Doubleday.

Huxley, J. (1970). *Memoirs.* London, England: George Allen & Unwin.

Juda, A. (1949). Relations between highest mental capacity and psychic abnormalities. *American Journal of Psychiatry, 106,* 296–307.

John, A. (1975). *Autobiography.* London, England: Jonathan Cape.

Lehmann, J. (1969). *In my own time: Memoirs of a literary life.* Boston: Little, Brown.

Lodge, H. (1975). *Early memories.* New York: Arno Press.

Martineau, H. (1969). *Harriet Martineau's autobiography.* Berlin: Gregg International.

McCurdy, H. (1960) The childhood pattern of genius, *Horizon, 2,* 33–38.

Mead, M. (1972). *Blackberry winter: My earlier years.* New York: William Morrow.

Meir, G. (1976). *My life.* London: Cox & Wyman.

Mill, J.S. (1963). *Autobiography.* (H.J. Laski, Ed.) London: Oxford University Press.

Miller, H. (1889). *Schools and schoolmasters.* Edinburgh: W. P. Nimmo, Hay & Mitchell.

Mitroff, I. (1974). Norms and counternorms in a select group of Apollo moon scientists. *American Sociological Review, 39,* 579–595.

Monroe, M. (1974). *My story.* New York: Stein & Day.

Moses, A. (1952). *Grandma Moses: My life's history* (Otto Kallir, Ed.). New York: Harper.

Mosley, S.O. (1968). *My life.* London, England: Thomas Nelsen.

Murphy, G., Murphy, L., & Newcomb, T. (1937). *Experimental social psychology.* New York: Harper.

Narayan, R. (1974). *My days.* New York: Viking Press.

Neill, A.S. (1972). *Neill Neill Orange Peel: An autobiography of the headmaster of Summerhill School.* New York: Hart.

O'Faolain, S. (1967). *Vive moi!* London, England: Rupert Hart-Davis Ltd.

Pritchett, V.S. (1968). *A cab at the door: An autobiography: Early years.* London, England: Chatto & Windus.

Robinson, E. (1973). *All my yesterdays.* New York: Hawthorn Books.

Roe, A. (1951a). A psychosocial study of eminent biologists. *Psychological Monographs, 65,* 1–68.

Roe, A. (1951b). A psychological study of eminent physical scientists. *Genetic Psychology Monographs, 43,* 121–235.

Rubinstein, A. (1973). *My young years.* New York: Knopf.

Sand, G. (1978). *My convent life* (M. E. McKay, Trans.). Chicago: Cassandra Editions (Original work published 1923)

Sternberg, R., & Davidson, J. (1986). Conceptions of giftedness: A map of the terrain. In R. Sternberg & J. Davidson (Eds.), *Conceptions of giftedness* (pp. 3–18). Cambridge, England: Cambridge University Press.

Taylor, A., Robinson, R., & McCormick, I. (1986). Written personal narratives as research documents: A case for their restoration. *International Review of Applied Psychology, 35,* 197–208.

Thackeray, W. (1978). *Memoirs of a Victorian gentleman.* London, England: Secker & Warburg.

Ustinov, P. (1977). *Dear me.* London, England: Heinemann.

Walberg, H., Rasher, S., & Hase, K. (1978). IQ correlates with high eminence. *The Gifted Child Quarterly,* 22, 196–200.

Walberg, H., Tsai, S., Weinstein, T., Gabriel, C., Rasher, S., Rosecrans, T., Rovai, E., Ide, J., Trujillo, M., R., & Vukosavich, P. (1981). Childhood traits and environmental conditions of highly eminent adults. *Gifted Child Quarterly,* 25, 103–107.

Waters, E. (1951). *His eye is on the sparrow.* New York: Doubleday.

Waugh, E. (1976). *The diaries of Evelyn Waugh.* London: Weidenfeld & Nicholson.

Williams, E. (1961). *George: An early autobiography.* London: Hamish Hamilton.

Williams, T. (1975). *Memoirs.* New York: Doubleday.

Wolf, T. (1973). *Alfred Binet.* Chicago: University of Chicago Press.

Woolf, L. (1970). *Sowing: An autobiography of the years 1880 to 1904.* London: Hogarth.

Zhukov, M. (1971). *The memoirs of Marshal Zhukov.* New York: Delacorte Press.

Zorach, W. (1967). *Art is my life.* Cleveland: World.

4
The Portrayal of Brightness in Children's Literature

WITH KEVIN MURPHY

Like any other minority group, gifted children may be deeply affected by the attitudes of the majority toward them. In fact, the image of giftedness conveyed in the media and in literature could conceivably have as great an impact on peer acceptance of the gifted as portrayals of racial and ethnic groups have on their members' welfare, since such attitudes toward brightness are imparted to children as early as attitudes toward any other group or characteristic.

Although stereotypic biases toward intellectual giftedness appear to be fairly common, there has been very little systematic study of adults' or children's attitudes toward brightness or creativity. As noted in Chapter 1, "egghead" stereotypes have at times pervaded the adult political scene. Such caricatures are also quite frequent in films aimed at the burgeoning adolescent market. However, these attitudes need not necessarily be negative. For example, observant Jewish families are required to tell the story of the Passover holiday to their children. A reference to four sons appears near the beginning of the prescribed text: one wise son, one wicked son, one simple son, and one who is too young to ask about the holiday. Suggestions are given as to how the three others might be handled, but the wise son is assigned the distinction of learning all about the festival.

Children's stories are an embodiment of the values, precepts, and prejudices of a society. In addition, these stories can play an important role in shaping children's developing beliefs and attitudes. If a negative image of a particular subgroup is portrayed in children's stories, the retelling of the stories will tend to perpetuate such images. While the immediate impact of the printed page may be less salient than that of television or film, books may play a unique role in the preservation and transmission of cultural attitudes. In contrast with today's television shows, which tend to be popular for a brief period, some children's stories have survived hundreds of years and myriads of technological innovations to be retold to generations of children.

Since children's literature appears to have the potential to influence the early attitudes of each new generation, it is not surprising that several previous researchers have considered the potential impact of children's literature. Perhaps the best-known psychological study of children's stories is MacLelland's (1961) analysis of the achievement motive in stories from various countries. He examined primers from 40 countries over two time periods and found that the achievement content therein was related to certain indices of economic growth. Stone (1978) and Taylor (1958) also analyzed children's stories for depictions of childhood, family relations, and child-rearing practices. More recently, a number of researchers have studied the portrayal of female characters and members of minority racial and ethnic groups in children's literature (Rogers, 1982).

Rogers (1982), in tracing the history of the systematic psychological study of children's fiction, noted that the major challenge in using children's stories in psychological studies is, as she put it, "turning 'soft' data into 'hard' data" (p. 47), that is, establishing means of reliably quantifying and analyzing this type of data. This is not surprising, because children's stories are subjective to begin with. Thus, the first challenge in assessing attitudes toward intellectual giftedness was to develop a meaningful and reliable system for identifying and coding such portrayals.

Development of Our Coding Manual

We discovered that books intended for preschoolers rarely contained any explicit depiction of the characters' intellect. Therefore, we decided to limit our sampling to stories written for school-age children. Our pilot analysis of several popular examples of children's fiction indicated that the intellectual abilities of many if not most characters were conveyed more or less directly. This made it possible to develop coding criteria that required minimal inference on the part of the raters. This was essential, since it would have been impossible to establish a reliable rating scheme if we were to permit coding of the characters' brightness based on the readers' own subjective impressions. For this reason our final procedures manual explicitly instructed the coders to rate the characters' intellectual abilities solely on the basis of descriptors contained in the text and to carefully record the descriptors that helped determine their ratings. "High" intelligence was to be coded if the characters or their actions were clearly described as smart, clever, or inventive, without any descriptors implying stupidity. When mixed descriptors were used, the character was to be rated as of "moderate or mixed" intellectual ability. "Low" ability was to be coded when a character or his or her behavior was clearly described as dumb, stupid, or forgetful, in the absence of any accompanying positive descriptions of cognitive ability. Characters could also be coded as "neutral" when there was no information available as to their intellectual ability.

The next coding category was the depicted evaluation of the character's intelligence. Coders were instructed to rate the author's evaluation of the characters' intellect specifically and not any evaluation of the person as a whole. Thus, a "positive" evaluation was coded when the characters' intelligence (or use of intelligence) was described in positive terms (e.g., "wonderfully smart"), was positively regarded by others, or led to positive consequences. Conversely, a "negative" evaluation was coded when the characters' intelligence was negatively regarded, described in negative terms, or led to negative outcomes within the story. Inconsistent or ambivalent evaluations of intelligence were coded as "mixed." "Neutral" was coded when no evaluation of the characters' intellect was apparent.

Whenever a character was coded as having high intelligence, that character's sociability was also coded. Again, sociability was coded according to specific descriptors provided, not necessarily the character's role in the plot. "Positive sociability" was coded when the character had many friends, was described as friendly or sociable, and/or had few difficulties with others. Conversely, "negative sociability" was coded when the character was described as a "loner," having few friends or having considerable difficulty with others. "Mixed" or "neutral" sociability ratings were used as indicated.

In addition to the portrayal of the characters' brightness, we were also interested in the depiction of intellectual activity in the stories. There were two types of activity that were coded as intellectual. The first involved tasks clearly associated with school, such as in-class work, homework, and projects. The second type of activity coded consisted of out-of-school intellectual pursuits such as reading, exploring, or experimenting *solely* for the purpose of increasing one's knowledge. Once identified, the evaluation of the intellectual activity contained in the stories was coded as positive, negative, mixed, or neutral. "Positive" was coded when the academic activity led to positive consequences, was positively regarded by the character, or described in positive terms. A "negative" evaluation was coded when such activity led to negative consequences, was negatively regarded by the character, or described in negative terms. A "mixed" evaluation was coded when both positive and negative descriptors were associated with such activity. Finally, when no evaluation of the intellectual activity was presented, "neutral" evaluation was coded.

In the original coding procedure, a separate category was used for "clever" acts. However, this category was eliminated because the clever acts were almost always executed by characters of high intelligence, making this category redundant. Furthermore, the interrater reliability for clever acts was slightly lower than for the other categories.

Only major characters were coded. These included main and support characters. A main character generally narrated the story. Multiple coding of main characters was permitted only if the story revolved equally around all of them. Support characters had to be present for most of the story, or play an important role, but were not the main characters. Peripheral characters were not coded.

Sampling Procedure

The 14th edition of the *Children's Catalogue* (Isaacson & Bogart, 1981), as well as the yearly supplements for 1982–1986, were used for the initial data pool. This catalogue is prepared for the guidance of children's libraries and retail bookshops and used by them as a guide in purchasing books for children's sections. There were approximately 2,000 entries in this preliminary data pool. From these, a sample of 50 was generated by selecting every 40th book from the alphabetical listing. Where the book selected was not available at the Ottawa Public Library, the next available book in the catalogue was substituted.

Reliability of Ratings

The books were coded by a research assistant with extensive background in English literature. Prior to coding, a number of books randomly selected from the library shelf were used for purposes of training the coder. These were coded by a second research assistant as well. The coding of the actual sample began after the first coder was trained to a prespecified criterion, which was set at interrater agreement exceeding 80% on all categories.

Reliability checks were conducted during the coding on a random sample of 13 of the 50 books coded in the study, or 25%. Interrater agreement by category averaged 83%, ranging from 78% for "clever acts" to 88% for level of intelligence. As mentioned above, the category of "clever acts" was subsequently eliminated. Thus, the average level of agreement was slightly higher than 84% for the categories included in the final quantitative analysis.

Quantitative Results: Portrayal of "Bright" Characters

There were a total of 120 major characters in the 50 books scanned. It was possible to code the intellectual level of 92 of these 120 major characters. Of these 92, 66 were coded as being of high intelligence, 11 as moderate, and 15 of low intellectual ability.

Positive descriptors were usually assigned to story characters of high intellectual ability. "Positive evaluation" was coded for 40 of the 66 "bright" characters (61%) while only nine of these characters were depicted negatively (the remaining 14 were coded as neutral or mixed). In contrast, 11 of the 15 characters of low intellectual ability were portrayed negatively. None had their low intelligence positively evaluated. Thus, it would appear that the stories as sampled contained a strong positive bias toward intellectual giftedness.

Since it was possible that the evaluation of intellectual activity might vary with the gender of the character, the analyses presented above were repeated for males and females separately. Eighty of the 120 characters coded were male. Of these, 42 were coded as being of high intelligence, 12 as being of low intellectual ability. Approximately 60% of the bright male characters ($n = 25$) were positively portrayed; only six were depicted negatively. Of the 40 female characters, 24 (60%) were coded as of high intellectual ability; three were coded as of low intelligence. Of the 24 bright female characters, 15 (or 63%) were positively depicted; three were assigned negative descriptors. Thus, it appeared that the tendency toward positively evaluating high intelligence did not depend on whether the character was male or female.

In contrast to the generally positive depicition of giftedness in these stories, our coding of the characters' sociability yielded very different findings. Of the 66 "bright" characters, only 10 (15%) were coded as highly sociable or socially interested. Over twice that many, 22 (33%) were coded as unsociable or not socially interested. Almost half of the 30 bright characters whose intelligence had been positively evaluated were coded as not socially interested or involved.

Of the 120 major characters, 30 conveyed some evaluation of intellectual activity out of school. Of the 30 evaluations, 19 were positive, including 13 of the 22 statements made by bright characters. There were only three negative evaluations of out-of-school intellectual activity in the stories studied. Thus, while the characters in these stories were not predominantly concerned with intellectual activity per se, when such activity was presented, it was, in general, positively evaluated.

A total of 34 of the major characters also conveyed some evaluation of the worth of school. Of these 34 evaluations, only 12 were positive, whereas 10 were negative. Of the 16 statements about school made by bright characters, 7 were positive, 3 were negative, 6 were ambivalent or mixed. Thus, school was not viewed as positively as learning in the more abstract sense. Furthermore, bright characters did not convey a more positive attitude toward school learning than did less intelligent characters.

In summary, brightness was generally portrayed in a positive light in contemporary children's fiction. There were no significant differences between the proportions of males and females depicted as bright, or in the authors' evaluations of the abilities of males or females. Most importantly, the bright characters basically appeared to be accepted as they were, even though they were not portrayed as highly interested or involved in social relations. Finally, intellectual activity and curiosity for its own sake were in general evaluated quite positively, whereas school-based learning received a much more mixed evaluation.

Qualitative Interpretation

A more qualitative interpretation of the stories scanned yields further insight into the portrayal of intellectual giftedness. First of all, brightness or intellect was rarely the central issue in a story. Although intellect was seen as a basically positive attribute, the bright characters and their intellectual strengths were not treated worshipfully or reverently. Some examples may be helpful in depicting this rather balanced portrayal of brightness in children's fiction, as well as the range of the connotations placed on intellect.

Intelligence as an Asset

Some of the stories portrayed learning and knowledge as an unqualified attribute. For example, H.M. Hoover's *Treasures of Morrow* (1976) is about two gifted children, Tia and Rabbit, who have fled their homeland to live in a more advanced society, Morrow. They had been born into a rather backward culture, consisting of people who had survived what we assume was a nuclear holocaust. The new society to which Tia and Rabbit now belong is made up of highly intelligent people who are the offspring of scientists who had predicted the nuclear disaster and made the necessary arrangements to survive. Tia and Rabbit are the products of a union between a scientist of the intellectual society and a woman from the backward one. These two children have the ability for mental telepathy, and they are rejected by their homeland. The people of Morrow, the advanced society, pick up their distress signals and rescue them. Upon arrival in Morrow, Tia remarks that there is a great deal she will have to learn. Both Tia and Rabbit are consistently described as highly intelligent. They are accepted in one society for their intellect, rejected in another—as may be the case for some real-life gifted children. Importantly, this book presents the attitudes of the backward society as negative and closed minded. In *Treasures of Morrow*, brightness as a trait is related to society's very survival.

A similar theme occurs in Alexander Key's (1965) *The Forgotten Door*. However, this time the less advanced society is the planet Earth. This book is about a boy from another world, Jon, who somehow slips through a forgotten door to Earth. His world is far more advanced than ours, and he has mental and physical capabilities far superior to those of Earthlings. However, on Earth, his abilities arouse suspicion, for "he sounds entirely too clever to be up to any good" (p. 99). Finally, he meets one understanding family, who appreciate his abilities and help him escape back to his own planet, where there are no laws, no leaders, and no wars, just intelligent "human" beings. Key portrays a fear of bright people here on Earth, but implies that if everyone were as gifted as Jon, the world would be a much better place.

In Frances Hodgson Burnett's *Sara Crewe* (1981), intellect restores grace to Cinderella-like Sara. Sara was put into a posh boarding school by her rich father, where, despite a certain oddness, she is treated admirably, until it is discovered that her father has died and left her penniless. The cruel schoolmistress then puts her to work as a servant. However, because she is bright, she is eventually adopted by an Indian gentleman who lives next door.

Intellect is admired even by ex-convicts in Patricia Beatty's *Jonathan Down Under* (1982). This book is about a boy who leaves America with his father in search of better opportunities. They end up in Australia during the Gold Rush. Jonathan, an intelligent child, learns a lot about his father and about life in general. When his father dies, Jonathan is left to fend for himself. He befriends two ex-convicts and helps them to strike it rich. The ex-cons admire him because of his intelligence and courage. They remark that "it is a sharp head, and courage, not size, that will take ye very far indeed" (p. 210).

Johanna Spyri's heroine *Heidi* (1959) is brought to live with her eccentric, recluse grandfather after her parents are killed. Heidi and her grandfather learn to love each other dearly and regret being separated when a relative takes Heidi to help care for an invalid girl. Heidi pines away for her grandfather, and they are reunited. Heidi and her grandfather are described as quite bright. Throughout, there is an emphasis on learning, especially on Heidi and Peter learning to read. Heidi is portrayed as very sociable and loved by everybody. Although the grandfather is also portrayed as intelligent, he is a loner. In the end, however, his relationship with Heidi changes him, and he becomes sociable, too.

Intelligence and Solitude

Other stories sampled also appeared to draw the association between high intelligence and a more solitary life-style. For instance, in *Bambi*, Bambi and his entire family (Salten, 1929) are all described as very clever, especially Bambi's mentor, the wise Old Stag. When young, Bambi seems to have been quite popular. However, according to the rather solitary old Stag, as one grows older, survival depends on wisdom, which is obtained by living alone: "to obtain wisdom, you have to live alone." As Bambi grows older, he too becomes more reclusive.

Eleanor Cameron's *A Room Made of Windows* (1971) is about Julia, whose mother is remarrying. Together they move to a new city. Leslie, described as a prodigy, is a girl who lives in Julia's new neighborhood. In contrast, Julia refrains from public displays of her knowledge, "I couldn't say 'pejorative' at school. They'd think I was showing off. Sometimes they think that anyway" (1971, p. 65). Leslie befriends Julia's brother, Greg, who is described as very studious. Greg's mother offered him the opportunity of inviting his own friends to their home. However, he could not, because he did not have many friends. His social isolation is attributed to his long periods of studying alone in his room.

Intellect as a Mixed Blessing

The well-known classic *Peter Pan* (Barrie, 1911) contains a more mixed depiction of intellect. Brightness here has much less to do with the outcome of the story. The hero, Peter, is portrayed as wise ("brilliant," p. 42, "frightfully cunning," p. 34, "clever," p. 42), but somewhat conceited. He is clearly well liked and wins out over the villainous Captain Hook. The wicked Captain Hook, however, is portrayed as a "brilliant" (p. 156) "mastermind genius" (p. 130). Thus, in *Peter Pan*, intellect is a quality that can lead to the accomplishment of great feats, both evil and benign. It is either a positive or negative feature, depending on the values and character of those who use it.

Divergent evaluations of brightness are also evident in Barbara Girion's *A Handful of Stars* (Girion, 1983). This story centers around Julie, a girl who develops epilepsy. Julie's sister, Nancy, is portrayed as being gifted. Nancy is quite popular; she is the captain of the cheerleaders, described explicitly as "a terrific person" (p. 92). Her giftedness is regarded positively by other story characters and by the author. Larry is Julie's classmate. He is described as "a great brain" (p. 19). Larry's mocking classmates consider him a "nerd" (p. 100), with whom they "would not be caught dead" (p. 46). The mixed message about brightness in *A Handful of Stars* is quite clear: Brightness is accepted if accompanied by other valued traits; "bookishness" is not.

Dorothy Crayder's *She, the Adventuress* (1973) is a tale about Maggie and Jasper, both intelligent children. Maggie is on a transatlantic voyage to visit a relative in Europe. Maggie is portrayed as popular. Jasper stows away aboard the ship to escape his family, who treat him as an outcast. They don't understand his intelligence. Together, Maggie and Jasper help, unwittingly, to capture an international art thief. Jasper initially perceives himself to be a social failure. In the end, he realizes that the only place he doesn't fit in is his family.

Rejection Because of Brightness

Although giftedness received a positive portrayal in most of the stories, this literature is not totally devoid of the "nerd" stereotype. Joan Aiken's *The Shadow Guests* (1980) is about Cosmo, who is sent to England to live with his aunt after his parents die. He finds out that a curse has been passed on to his family. The firstborn son will die tragically, and the mother will then die of grief. Cosmo sets out to stop the curse, and in doing so meets members of his family from ancient times. Much of the story takes place in Cosmo's new school. There he is made fun of because of his foreign ways and because of his brightness. In the end, Cosmo is befriended by two other bright children.

Another example of peer rejection of the gifted is contained in Ursula K. LeGuin's *Very Far Away From Anywhere Else* (1976). This book is about Owen, a high school student who is very unpopular. Even his parents do not understand him. He becomes friendly with a fellow student named Natalie. The story then concentrates on the development of their friendship and the maturing effects it has on both of them. Owen is characterized as highly intelligent and as a total social reject. Only Natalie will accept him as he is. Owen notes that:

...No matter how I tried, I was never going to be an extrovert, or popular, or one of the group. (p. 32)
...I was the kind of person that just does not fit into this kind of society. What should they like me for, my brain? Nobody likes brains. (LeGuin, 1976, p. 39)

Conclusion

It should be noted that the above examples were selected because they seemed most relevant to the topic of the portrayal of giftedness and illustrated the range of such portrayals. However, not all of the stories sampled dealt as explicitly with the issue of giftedness. Many of the stories scanned contained no more than fleeting reference to the characters' intelligence.

Interestingly, the authors of children's fiction seem to have intuitively recapitulated the picture of the peer acceptance of the gifted that has emerged from theory (Chapter 1) and research (Chapter 2). The gifted are basically well accepted, with some notable exceptions. Where a highly intelligent character was negatively portrayed, this tended to relate to accompanying devalued nonintellective attributes, such as physical clumsiness. Such qualifications to the acceptance of gifted adolescents have been prominently noted in the giftedness literature (Tannenbaum, 1962). A child who sampled this literature would probably not be subjected to substantial distortions about bright people. As depicted, intellect is an asset in life, but one that is more valued in certain settings than others. Wisdom can be put to good use, but can also be, on occasion, misdirected. Those endowed with such gifts may withdraw from social interaction at times in order to cultivate their talents.

If our children's stories are a statement of our society's values, what do they say about our perceptions of the gifted? In all fairness, we must conclude that this source does not indicate that giftedness is a matter of overriding concern in the minds of our storytellers. However, when they do address this issue, they seem to deal with it realistically.

At the same time, we must ask ourselves whether children's stories are an adequate reflection of the values and beliefs of society as a whole. While the proportion of children who have access to this body of literature is surely greater today than in previous centuries (see Rogers, 1982 for fuller discussion), there probably still are many children who receive minimal exposure to books. Furthermore, it has been documented that television and film reach a large segment of society. These media may therefore exert greater influence on people's attitudes than books do. It might be profitable to continue this exploration with an analysis of the portrayal of brightness in children's television shows and films. Finally, it is beyond the scope of this study to demonstrate a causal relationship between portrayals of giftedness in children's literature and public attitudes. However, what has been demonstrated is that intellectual giftedness is systematically portrayed in children's fiction. Since this portrayal seems positive, there would appear to be little grounds for implicating children's literature in the emergence of any negative stereotypes of the gifted child.

References

Aiken, J. (1980). *The shadow guests*. London: Jonathan Cape.

Barrie, J.M. (1911). *Peter Pan*. New York: Charles Scribner's Sons.

Beatty, P. (1982). *Jonathan down under*. New York: William Morrow.

Burnett, F.H. (1981). *Sara Crewe or whatever happened at Miss Minchin's*. New York: G.P. Putnam's Sons.

Cameron, E. (1971). *A room made of windows*. Boston: Little, Brown.

Crayder, D. (1973). *She, the adventuress*. New York: Atheneum.

Girion, B. (1983). *A handful of stars*. New York: Dell.

Hoover, H.M. (1976). *Treasures of Morrow*. New York: Four Winds Press.

Isaacson, R., & Bogart G. (1981). *The children's catalogue* (14th ed.). New York: H.W. Wilson.

Key, A. (1965). *The forgotten door*. Philadelphia: Westminster Press.

LeGuin, U.K. (1976). *Very far away from anywhere else*. New York: Atheneum.

MacLelland, D. (1961). *The achieving society*. Toronto: Van Nostrand.

Rogers, E. (1982). *Attitudes to children in English children's prose fiction, 1740–1840*. Unpublished doctoral dissertation, Carleton University, Ottawa Ontario, Canada.

Salten, F. (1929). *Bambi*. New York: Grosset & Dunlop.

Spyri, J. (1959). *Heidi*. New York: Franklin Watts.

Stone, L. (1978). *The family, sex and marriage in England, 1500–1800*. London: Weidenfeld & Nicholson.

Tannenbaum, A. (1962). *Adolescent attitudes toward academic brilliance*. New York: Teachers College Press.

Taylor, R. (1958). *The angel-makers: A study in the psychological origins of historical change*. London: Heinemann.

5
The Social Self-Concepts of Gifted Children: Delusions of Ungrandeur?

Probably no psychological construct has captured as much of the attention of both child psychologists and educators as self-concept. Concern for children's feelings about themselves is equally evident in volumes to be found on the shelves of popular bookstores. Self-concept has been seen as the core of human personality (Lecky, 1945). The emergence of positive self-concepts has also often been regarded as a major objective of the school system (Purkey, 1970). Given this emphasis, it is not surprising that the self-concept of the gifted child has been the subject of considerable speculation, numerous studies, and many remedial prescriptions. Tannenbaum (1986) noted that intelligence and self-concept are complementary in the ways that they facilitate the emergence of gifted behaviors. Arguing that a person with determination is more likely to succeed than one with ability, he presented self-concept and eminent accomplishments as something of a feedback loop. Those who *think* of themselves as gifted will try to act in ways that will bring their accomplishments in line with their self-images. In turn, these excellent achievements will further enhance the indivjdual's self-concept. If one accepts this argument, it is important to assess the relationship between self-concept and giftedness, since self-concept may serve as an important factor influencing how well gifted children attain their potential. This chapter is a critical summary of research on the self-concepts of the gifted, with emphasis on their social self-concepts. Throughout this review of the literature, repeated reference will be made to several recurrent issues in self-concept theory and measurement.

One Self-Concept or Many?

In contrast with the widespread consensus on the importance of self-concept, there is little agreement on the definition and conceptualization of this construct. In general terms, self-concept has been seen as individuals' perceptions of themselves. In specific terms, it is their feelings, attitudes, and knowledge about their abilities, skills, appearance, and social acceptability (Byrne, 1984; Labenne & Greene, 1969; West & Fish, 1973). Byrne's (1984) review outlines four possible models of self-concept. The first of these is the *nomothetic* position, which holds that self-concept is essentially a unidimensional phenomenon in which a fairly global or general self-concept can explain behavior in a great variety of settings and situations. The second theoretical position is that self-concept is hierarchical in nature. According to this position, there are multiple, separate facets of self-concept that can be ranked in hierarchical fashion (Shavelson & Bolus, 1982). Situation-specific self-concepts (e.g., academic self-concept, social self-concept) are at the base of the hierarchy, with the more stable general self-concept at the apex. In contrast, *taxonomic* models emphasize the separateness and situation specificity of the various facets of self-concept. Finally, *compensatory* models hold that there is an inverse relationship between the various aspects of self-concept. An individual low on one aspect (say, physical self-concept) might be compensated by elevations on other dimensions of self-concept (academic, social, or emotional).

Byrne (1984) concluded that, while no unidimensional model of self-concept has attained widespread acceptance, the multidimensional nature of self-concept has been amply demonstrated by factor analysis and related techniques. Winne and Marx (1981) noted that most prevailing models comprise three or four specific facets: academic, social, physical, and sometimes emotional. This multidimensionality is of primary importance when considering the self-concepts of gifted children. Intuitively, one would expect that most intellectually gifted children would have high academic self-concepts by virtue of their experiences of success in academic situations. If we accept that premise, separation of the academic dimension from the social, physical, and emotional is essential for a meaningful picture of the psychosocial adjustment of the gifted. In fact, the compensatory models might lead us to wonder if individuals with high levels of academic self-concept are not compensating for lower self-concepts in the other domains.

The Social Origin of Self-Concept

Theorists are nearly unanimous in their assumption that self-concept is of social origin (Epstein, 1973; Winne & Marx, 1981). Cooley (1902) and Harter (1983) introduced the concept of a "social mirror": our self-image is a reflection of the way we imagine others think of us. Adler implicated feelings of inferiority as the central driving force in personality dysfunction (Ansbacher & Ansbacher, 1956). Mead (1925) posited that individuals assume the basic attitude that others take toward them. If we accept these ideas uncritically, we might predict that gifted children would have average or above average social self-concepts. As detailed in Chapter 2, most studies have revealed that peers' perceptions of gifted children are positive.

Not all theorists, however, concur on the degree of the social origin of self-concept. In his discussions of the emergence of self-esteem, Piaget (1981) emphasized the dynamic interplay of the individual's processes of self-evaluation and the evaluations of that individual by others. He noted that one's self-esteem is not the sum total of evaluations by others. Once children achieve a certain maturity in cognitive development, they evaluate themselves continually. These self-evaluations occur independently of social relationships, invoking "an application of socially acquired behavior to the self" (Piaget, 1981, p. 49).

Furthermore, there are several reasons to believe that gifted children may be somewhat severe in their self-evaluations. One of these factors is their heightened sensitivity. This phenomenon is discussed by Freeman (1985). She points out that the child's hypersensitivity to sensory input may itself create intellectual giftedness by allowing the assimilation of massive amounts of sensory input. While this leaves the gifted child extraordinarily able to pick up communication signals, this hyperacute perception can also cause distortions of those signals. In her experience, this has meant that gifted children are more responsive than others to criticism, taking it very much to heart. Furthermore, their tendencies toward social isolation may restrict the flow of social messages, including statements that disconfirm any information that leads to self-devaluation. It should be noted that Ritchie, Bernard, and Shertzer (1982) failed to corroborate the view that the intellectually gifted display higher levels of interpersonal sensitivity than controls. In their study, 10 and 12 year olds were asked to perceive and differentiate the behavioral intentions of individuals involved in videotaped interpersonal vignettes.

Freeman (1985) also noted that the gifted child's perfectionism, perhaps born of more fine-tuned perceptions of objects, people, and relationships, can lead to further devaluations of self-concept. Developmental psychologists have identified stages in children's understanding of friendship (Selman, 1980). Imagine a not uncommon situation in which a researcher asks a group of children how many friends they have. The gifted participants, in addition to any other sources of distortion in their responses, may respond on the basis of a more sophisticated understanding of friendship. Many of the controls might be at a lower stage in the understanding of friendships and enumerate their immediate play companions without consideration of enduring relationship characteristics.

Leaders in educational programming for the gifted have identified other reasons for possible impairment of self-concept among this group of children. It has been noted that the gifted child is often aware of what *should* be done in a situation prior to having the resources to accomplish such ideal performance (Foster, 1985; Gowan, 1977). This would lead to inherent dissatisfaction with one's own social behavior. In addition, the gifted child's intellectual precocity and independence may be deceiving. They may deceive adults into thinking that the gifted child is equally mature in all respects. Acting on such outward appearances, adults may treat the gifted child as a fellow adult, and not provide necessary guidance, interpretation, reassurance, and support (Foster, 1985).

Review of Self-Concept Studies

Table 5.1 is a summary of known studies in which the general self-concept of gifted children is compared with controls. As shown, over half of the studies have found that the general self-concepts of gifted children are higher than that of the controls. In all the others, no significant differences were found between gifted and controls. Thus, while researchers are not consistent in demonstrating an advantage for gifted children in terms of global self-concept, there are no indications of any disadvantage for the gifted. At first glance, this picture of the self-concept of the gifted child appears to mirror the literature on their peer acceptance, reviewed in Chapter 2.

There are a number of methodological problems with many of these studies. First of all, several studies have compared self-concept scores of the gifted with the norms stated in the manuals for the standardization samples (Coleman & Fults, 1982; Ketcham & Snyder, 1977; Maddux et al.,

TABLE 5.1. Summary of studies comparing gifted and nongifted children on general self-concept.

Author (date)	Age range	Results
Klein & Cantor (1976)	K to grade 4	Probably NS[a]
Milgram & Milgram (1976)	Grades 4–8	+
Ketcham & Snyder (1977)	Grades 2–4	NS
O'Such, Havertape & Pierce (1979)	Ages 8–12	+
Stopper (1978/1979)	Grades 2, 4, and 6	NS
McQuilkin (1980/1981)	Grades 4–5	+
Tidwell (1980)	Grade 10	NS and +[b,c]
Bracken (1980)	Mean 9.8 years	NS[b]
Karnes & Wherry (1981)	Grades 4–7	+
Lehman & Erdwins (1981)	Grade 3	+
Coleman & Fults (1982)	Grades 4–6	Probably +[a,b]
Maddux, Scheiber, Bass (1982)	Grades 5–6	Probably +[a,b]
Winne, Woodlands, & Wong (1982)	Grades 4–7	NS
Janos, Fung, & Robinson (1985)	Ages 5–10	+[b]
Kelly & Colangelo (1985)	Grades 7–9	+
Holahan & Brounstein (1986)	Grade 7	NS

Note. + = gifted scored higher than controls; NS = no significant differences.
[a] No significance level reported.
[b] Comparison with standardization norms.
[c] Different results on two self-concept measures.

1982; Tidwell, 1980). While this is not without some value, it cannot be inferred from these studies that the self-concepts of gifted children are different from those of nongifted children in their own communities (see Chapter 2). Furthermore, these inferences cannot be of any greater value than the adequacy of the norming procedures and standardization samples of the respective instruments. As detailed in the following discussion, this is not a trivial concern.

Other studies have used control groups that may not be entirely comparable with the gifted group. Coleman and Fults (1982) compared the gifted with high-achieving normals. As in research on other implications of giftedness, inconsistent identification criteria make interpretation of several studies difficult. For example, Bracken's (1980) "gifted" subjects had IQs as low as 120, as did those in Karnes and Wherry's (1981) research. The criteria for identifying subjects as gifted were not specified in several studies (e.g., O'Such et al., 1979). Ketcham and Snyder's (1977) results may be qualified by the fact that the gifted participants in the study were of the uppermost socioeconomic levels and were enrolled in private school. These children's self-concepts may have been highly affected by environmental factors as well as intellectual precocity. While Winne et al. (1982) utilized both "normal" and learning disabled children as controls, only the differences between the gifted and learning disabled groups were included in the preplanned statistical contrasts subjected to analysis. It is not clear, therefore, whether those findings should be attributed to distortions of self-regard that accompany intellectual giftedness, learning disabilities, or both.

Domain-Specific Self-Concept Studies

The major limitation of the studies summarized in Table 5.1 is their failure to analyze self-concept by specific domain. This shortcoming alone is sufficient to question their value. Table 5.2 displays the results of studies that have compared gifted and nongifted children in terms of the various domains of self-concept previously discussed. It is apparent that the gifted child's commonly reported advantage in self-concept is probably limited to the academic domain. The findings of the half dozen studies summarized in Table 5.2 are strengthened by research by Ross and Parker (1980). While that study did not involve a "normal" control group, it was found that both gifted boys and girls displayed significantly higher academic than social self-concepts.

Sex Differences

Despite the many theoretical writings and case studies devoted to the self-concept of gifted females (e.g., Kerr, 1985), analyses of sex differences were reported in only a few of the studies. No sex differences were found by Karnes and Wherry (1981), whose self-concept measures were rather

TABLE 5.2. Studies comparing self-concepts of gifted and nongifted children, differentiated by self-concept domain.

Author (date)	Age range	Results
Academic self-concept		
Colangelo & Pfleger (1978)	Grades 9–12	Probably +[a]
Winne et al. (1982)	Grades 4–7	Probably NS[b,c]
Kelly & Colangelo (1985)	Grades 7–9	+
Holohan & Brounstein (1986)	Grade 7	+
Schneider et al. (1986)	Grades 5, 8, and 10	+
Physical self-concept		
Milgram & Milgram (1976)	Grades 4–8	–
Winne et al. (1982)	Grades 4–7	Probably NS[b,c]
Kelly & Colangelo (1985)	Grades 7–9	Probably NS[c]
Holohan & Brounstein (1986)	Grade 7	–
Schneider et al. (1986)	Grades 5, 8, and 10	NS
Social self-concept		
Milgram & Milgram (1976)	Grades 4–8	NS
Winne et al. (1982)	Grades 4–7	Probably NS[b,c]
Kelly & Colangelo (1985)	Grades 7–9	+
Holohan & Brounstein (1986)	Grade 7	–
Schneider et al. (1986)	Grades 5, 8, and 10	NS

Note. + = gifted scored higher than controls; – = gifted scored lower than controls; NS = no significant differences.
[a] In comparison with standardization norms.
[b] Comparison of gifted and "normal" groups (gifted vs. learning disabled comparisons also reported).
[c] No significance level reported.

global. A few sex differences were found in the more specific analyses conducted by Milgram and Milgram (1976). On some comparisons, gifted girls displayed higher self-concepts than gifted boys. There were also some interactive effects. Nongifted girls were found to be more anxious than nongifted boys; this finding did not hold for gifted subjects.

Sex differences in self-concept among gifted and control subjects in grades 5, 8, and 10 were explored by Schneider et al. (1986). There were no sex differences at the grade 5 level. At both the grade 8 and 10 levels, boys displayed higher general and physical self-concepts than girls, regardless of membership in the gifted or control groups; there were no sex differences on the academic or social self-concept scales.

Thus, the very limited data on sex differences in the self-concepts of gifted children are somewhat contradictory and inconclusive. Given the attention to self-concept in the literature on giftedness in women, it is important that future studies include analysis for gender differences.

Self-Concept of the Very Highly Gifted

As noted in Chapters 1 and 2, the social adjustment of the very highly gifted has been considered much more problematic than that of moderately gifted children. Janos (1983) systematically explored this possibility. He compared a group of 32 highly gifted elementary school-age children with 49 moderately gifted youngsters in terms of ratings on the Piers-Harris scale. Both groups far exceeded the normative means on the Piers-Harris. There was no significant difference between the scores of the highly gifted and moderately gifted. Unfortunately, Janos did not break down the ratings by self-concept domain. Future researchers may wish to conduct such domain-specific comparisons of the highly and moderately gifted in order to determine whether the social self-concepts of the highly gifted reflect the peer relations difficulties discussed in previous chapters.

Instrumentation

Self-concept measures have been widely criticized for their limited norms, lack of reliability, and poor validity data (Byrne, 1983; Lakey, 1977; Wylie, 1974). In many of the studies reported in this chapter, excessive confidence may have been placed in the psychometric properties of these measures. There is little awareness in this body of literature that these measures are not as extensively normed and validated as such mainstays as the Minnesota Multiphasic Personality Inventory (MMPI) or Wechsler scales.

Self-concept was measured by means of the Piers-Harris Children's Self-Concept Scale in the majority of studies (Karnes & Wherry, 1981; Ketcham & Snyder, 1977; Klein & Cantor, 1976; O'Such et al., 1979; McQuilkin, 1980/1981; Stopper, 1978/1979). There has also been some use of the Coopersmith Scale (e.g., Klein & Cantor, 1976; Winne et al., 1982). Harter (1983) reviewed the psychometric properties of these children's self-concept scales. While impressive test-retest and split-half reliability was reported for the Coopersmith inventory, there is some difficulty in defining the construct that is reliably measured. Harter attributed these validity problems to the fact that the Coopersmith is essentially a junior version of an adult self-concept scale. The Piers-Harris Scale is an improvement, in that the items derive from a pool of statements collected from children. The major limitation of the Piers-Harris is the fact that most users of the scale, including those indicated in Table 5.1, limit their analyses to the total self-concept score, ignoring the component factors that have emerged in factor analyses. By doing so, inferences can be made only about global self-concept, despite the fact that more meaningful data relative to the various facets of self-concept would be readily available within the same measure. Thus, most of the researchers whose work is summarized here have used a good instrument, but not made optimal use of it.

Comparison of Peer and Self-Evaluations

Attention is drawn to the differences between the results contained in Table 2.2, which summarized studies of the peer acceptance of the gifted, and the results pertaining to social self-concept in Table 5.2. It would appear very possible that while gifted children are generally well accepted by their peers, this acceptance is not fully reflected in their social self-concepts. If this phenomenon is verified, it would underscore Piaget's position, discussed previously, that an individual's self-image is not the mere reflection of the social messages received. Verification of this hypothesis would require systematic comparison of the peer acceptance and social self-concepts of the same persons.

The comparison of peer and self-evaluations of an individual's social competence is a complex undertaking. In general, the best way to compare two sources of information about the same psychological construct is to examine their concordance in rating the same behaviors (Campbell & Fiske, 1959). This method has at times been applied to children's social behavior. For example, a self-report scale has been developed to parallel the Pupil Evaluation Inventory, a popular peer nomination instrument (Pekarik, Prinz, Liebert, Weintraub, & Neale, 1976). However, such self-reports may not fully capture the essence of an individual's feelings of self-worth. Self-esteem is a private matter, built of thoughts and impressions that far transcend the rather concrete behaviors that peers are meaningfully able to observe and rate. Peers may not have access to many of the dimensions of social behavior that are woven into a person's social self-concept. There are other obstacles to the systematic comparison of self-concept and peer ratings. Asher (1986, personal communication) noted that the most socially competent individuals, out of modesty and their own exemplary social skills, may decline to rate their social relations as superlative.

Cognizant of these pitfalls, Schneider and co-workers (1986) compared the social self-concepts of gifted children in grades 5, 8, and 10, with peer nominations for sociability/leadership received by the same subjects. Their sampling procedure, sample size, and instrumentation are detailed in Chapter 2. Both the social self-concept scores and the peer nominations for social competence were divided into quintiles according to the distributions of these scores for the random control group subjects. It was predicted that each child's social self-concept score and peer nomination score would fall within the same quintile.

The frequencies of subjects' social self-concept scores falling within the same quintile, at least one quintile below, or one quintile above the prediction based on peer nominations were tabulated for both the gifted and control groups. These data are depicted pictorally in Figure 5.1. The proportions of scores falling below prediction within the gifted and control groups were compared by means of 2×3 chi-square analysis performed separately at each grade level. In grade 5, a significant disproportion ($p <$ .05) of gifted children displayed social self-perceptions below prediction. A nonsignificant trend in the same direction was observed in grade 8. In grade 10, the self-perceptions of gifted children with regard to social

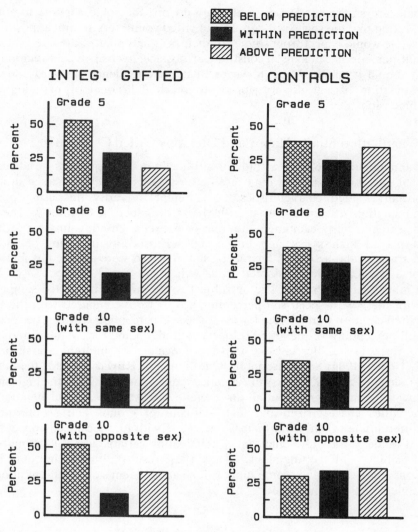

FIGURE 5.1. Self-ratings of social competence versus predictions made from peer ratings. From "Social Self-Concepts of Gifted Children: Delusions of Ungrandeur?" by B. Schneider, J. Ledingham, G. Crombie, and M. Clegg, paper presented at the 1986 meeting of the American Psychological Association.

competence in opposite-sex situations were disproportionately below pre-dicition. This disproportion achieved statistical significance ($p < .05$) for the entire grade 10 gifted sample, but was much more pronounced for gifted boys. The findings with regard to predicted self-perceptions of social competence in same-sex situations were nonsignificant. Although these data are somewhat inconsistent, they do provide some support for the position that the social self-concepts of gifted youngsters are not as positive as one would expect from studies of their peer acceptance. Lowered social self-perception can in itself constitute an obstacle to positive peer relations. It should be pointed out, however, that these tendencies toward underestimation of self do not appear to reach delusional or pathological dimensions.

What Differentiates Happy and Unhappy Gifted Children?

Tannenbaum (1962), in a study of attitudes toward brightness, predicted that gifted adolescents would fare better socially if they possessed other socially valued characteristics. An attempt to verify this using peer nominations (Schneider et al., 1986) was described in Chapter 2. These researchers also examined differences between gifted youngsters who displayed high social and low social self-concepts in terms of their extracurricular activities. Extracurricular interests were assessed by means of a self-report scale adopted from Achenbach and Edelbrock's (1978) Child Behavior Profile. The 69 subjects (one third of the gifted sample) with the lowest social self-perception scores were compared with the 67 gifted children who had the lowest social self-perception scores. The social self-perceptions of the gifted subjects in grades 5 and 8 were measured by Harter's (1982) Perceived Competence Scale for Children. Marsh and O'Neill's (1984) Self-Description Questionnaire III was used for the 10th grade participants. There were significant differences between the high and low self-concept groups at all three age levels. At grades 5 and 10, sports activities characterized the high self-concept groups and significantly differentiated them from their counterparts with low social self-concepts. At grade 8, the only significant discriminating variable was self-ratings of sociability and "getting along." Thus, these results, although not entirely consistent, do provide some support for Tannenbaum's observations about athletic activity and giftedness.

Creativity and Self-Concept

In virtually all the studies discussed, the gifted samples were defined on the basis of individual or group IQ scores. There has been comparatively little study of the self-concepts of children with other than "schoolhouse" giftedness (see Chapter 1). Wallach and Kogan (1965) conducted a now classic study of the self-concept of highly creative young children. They found that youngsters who scored high in *both* intelligence and creativity were also high in self-confidence and self-esteem. This did not apply to the more obstreperous group of participants who were high in creativity but scored low on measures of intelligence. Although extreme caution must be exercised in generalizing results from adults to children, mention should be made of some recurring patterns in the adult research relevant to the self-esteem of creative individuals. Rather consistently, they have been found to be self-reliant and self-accepting, although socially introverted (Barron & Harrington, 1981). Further research is necessary before these traits can be responsibly attributed to creative children.

Conclusion

While many references are made to the superior self-concept of the gifted child, these may involve an overgeneralization of the available results. There has been relatively little domain-specific research on the self-concept of the gifted child. Those domain-specific studies strongly suggest that the gifted child's advantage in self-concept over nongifted counterparts is limited to the academic domain. When results specific to the social self-concepts of gifted children are considered, it appears quite possible that their internal representations of their social behavior do not fully reflect the rather optimistic picture of peer acceptance that has emerged in the studies summarized in Chapter 2. Furthermore, there are few conclusive data available regarding the self-concepts of highly creative children or youngsters with other types of specific talents. Furthermore, there has been relatively little research on the self-concept of the one-in-a-thousand genius, as opposed to the uppermost 2% or 3% of the population usually enrolled in special school programs. Further exploration is needed to corroborate case study data regarding sex differences in the self-concepts of gifted children.

References

Achenbach, T.M., & Edelbrock, C.S. (1978). The classification of child psycho-pathology: A review and analysis of empirical efforts. *Psychological Bulletin* 1978, *85*, 1275–1301.

Ansbacher, H., & Ansbacher, R. (1956). *The individual psychology of Alfred Adler.* New York: Harper.

Barron, F.X., & Harrington, D. (1981). Creativity, intelligence and personality. *Annual Review of Psychology, 32,* 439–476.

Bracken, B. (1980). Comparison of self-attitudes of gifted children and children in a nongifted, normative group. *Psychological Reports, 47,* 715–718.

Byrne, B.M. (1983). Investigating measures of self-concept. *Measurement and Evaluation in Guidance, 16,* 115–126.

Byrne, B.M. (1984). The general/academic self-concept nomological network: A review of construct validation research. *Review of Educational Research, 54,* 427–456.

Campbell, D., & Fiske, D.W. (1959). Convergent and discriminant validation by the multitrait-multimethod matrix. *Psychological Bulletin, 56,* 81–105.

Coleman, J., & Fults, B. (1982). Self-concept and the gifted classroom: The role of social comparisons. *Gifted Child Quarterly, 26,* 116–120.

Colangelo, N., & Pfleger, L. (1978). Academic self-concept of gifted high school students. In N. Colangelo & R. Zaffran (Eds.), *New voices in counseling the gifted* (pp. 188–193). Dubuque IA: Kendall/Hunt.

Cooley, C. (1902). *Human nature and the social order.* New York: Scribners.

Epstein, S. (1973). The self-concept revisited: Or a theory of a theory. *American Psychologist, 28,* 404–416.

Foster, W. (1985). Helping a child toward individual excellence. In J. Feldhusen (Ed.), *Toward excellence in gifted education* (pp. 135–161). Denver: Love.

Freeman, J. (1985). Emotional aspects of giftedness. In J. Freeman (Ed.), *The psychology of gifted children* (pp. 247–264). New York: Wiley.

Gowan, J.C. (1977). Background and history of the gifted child movement. In J.C. Stanley, W.C. George, & C.H. Solano (Eds.), *The gifted and the creative: A fifty year perspective* (pp. 5–27). Baltimore: Johns Hopkins.

Harter, S. (1982). The perceived competence scale for children. *Child Development, 53,* 87–97.

Harter, S. (1983). Developmental perspectives on the self-system. In P. Mussen (Ed.), *Handbook of child psychology* (Vol. 4, Socialization, Personality and Social Development pp. 275–386). New York: Wiley.

Holahan, W., & Brounstein, P. (1986, August). *The relationships between domains of self-concept and attributional patterns in academically gifted and competent adolescents.* Paper presented at the meeting of the American Psychological Association, Washington, DC.

Janos, P.M. (1983). The psychosocial adjustment of children of very superior intellectual ability. *Dissertation Abstracts International, 44,* 1030A. (University Microfilms No. DA 8318378).

Janos, P.M., Fung, H., & Robinson, N.M. (1985). Perceptions of deviation and self-concept within an intellectually gifted sample. *Gifted Child Quarterly, 29,* 78–82.

Karnes, F.A., & Wherry, G.N. (1981). Self-concepts of gifted students as measured by the Piers-Harris self-concept scale. *Psychological Reports, 49,* 903–906.

Kelly, K., & Colangelo, N. (1985). Academic and social self-concepts of gifted, general and special students. *Exceptional Children, 50,* 551–554.

Kerr, B.A. (1985). *Smart girls, gifted women.* Columbus: Ohio Psychology Publishing.

Ketcham, B., & Snyder, R. (1977). Self-attitudes of the intellectually and socially advantaged student: Normative study of the Piers-Harris children's self-concept scale. *Psychological Reports, 40,* 111–116.

Klein, P., & Cantor, L. (1976). Gifted children and their self-concept. *Creative Child and Adult Quarterly, 1,* 98–101.

Labenne, W., & Greene, B. (1969). *Educational implications of self-concept theory.* Pacific Palisades, CA: Goodyear.

Lakey, J. (1977). *A multitrait, multimethod validation of measures of student school self-concept and attitude toward school in second and third grade children.* Unpublished doctoral dissertation. California State University at Long Beach.

Lecky, P. (1945). *Self-consistency: A theory of personality.* New York: Island.

Lehman, E., & Erdwins, E. (1981). The social and emotional adjustment of young, intellectually gifted children. *Gifted Child Quarterly, 25,* 134–137.

Maddux, C., Scheiber, L., & Bass, J. (1982). Self-concept and social distance in gifted chldren. *Gifted Child Quarterly, 26,* 77–81.

Marsh, H., & O'Neill, R. (1984). Self-Description Questionnaire III: The construct validity of multidimensional self-concept ratings by late adolescents. *Journal of Educational Measurement, 21,* 153–174.

Marx, R., & Winne, P. (1980). Self-concept validation research: Some current complex ties. *Measurement and Evaluation in Guidance, 13,* 72–82.

McQuilkin, C.E. (1980/1981). A comparison of personal and social concepts of gifted elementary school students in different school programs. *Dissertation Abstracts International, 41,* 3530A. (University Microfilms No. 810704)

Mead, G. (1925). The genesis of the self and social control. *International Journal of Ethics, 35,* 251–273.

Milgram, R.M., & Milgram, N.A. (1976). Personality characteristics of gifted Israeli children. *Journal of Genetic Psychology, 129,* 185–194.

O'Such, T., Havertape, J., & Pierce, K. (1979). Group differences in self-concept among handicapped, normal and gifted learners. *Humanist Educator, 18,* 15–22.

Pekarik, E., Prinz, R., Liebert, D., Weintraub, S., & Neale, J. (1976). The pupil evaluation inventory: A sociometric technique for assessing children's social behavior. *Journal of Abnormal Child Psychology, 4,* 83–97.

Piaget, J. (1981). *Intelligence and affectivity: Their relationship during child development.* T.A. Brown & C.E. Kaegi (Trans. & Eds.). Palo Alto, CA: Annual Reviews. (Original work published 1954.)

Purkey, W. (1970). *Self-concept and school achievement.* Englewood Cliffs, NJ: Prentice-Hall.

Ritchie, A., Bernard, J., & Shertzer, B. (1982). A comparison of academically talented children and academically average children on interpersonal sensitivity. *Gifted Child Quarterly, 26,* 105–109.

Ross, A., & Parker, M. (1980). Academic and social self-concepts of the academically gifted. *Exceptional Children, 47,* 6–10.

Schneider, B.H., Clegg, M.R., Byrne, B.M., Ledingham, J.E., & Crombie, G. (1986). *The social consequences of giftedness in Ontario schools.* Unpublished research report, Social Sciences and Humanities Research Council of Canada and Ontario Ministry of Education.

Selman, R. (1980). *The growth of interpersonal understanding.* Orlando, FL: Academic Press.

Shavelson, R., & Bolus, R. (1982). Self-concept: The interplay of theory and methods. *Journal of Educational Psychology, 74,* 3–17.

Stopper, C.J. (1978/1979). The relationships of the self-concept of gifted and non-gifted elementary school students to achievement, sex, grade level and membership in a self-contained academic program for the gifted. (Doctoral dissertation, University of Pennsylvania). *Dissertation Abstracts International, 40,* 90A. (University Microfilms No. 79-11905)

Tannenbaum, A.J. (1962). *Adolescent attitudes towards academic brilliance.* New York: Teachers College Press.

Tannenbaum, A.J. (1986). Giftedness: A psychosocial approach. In R. Sternberg

& J. Davidson (Eds.), *Conceptions of giftedness* (pp. 21–52). Cambridge, England: Cambridge University Press.

Tidwell, R. (1980). a psycho-educational profile of 1,593 gifted high school students. *Gifted Child Quarterly, 24,* 63–68.

Wallach, M., & Kogan, N. (1965). *Modes of thinking in young children.* New York: Holt, Rinehart & Winston.

West, C., & Fish, J. (1973). *Reslationship between self-concept and school achievement: A survey of empirical investigations.* University of Illinois, Urbana-Champaign (ERIC Document Reproduction Service No. ED092 239).

Winne, P., & Marx, R. (1981, March). *Convergent and discriminant validity in self-concept measurement.* Paper presented at the meeting of the American Educational Association, Los Angeles.

Winne, P., Woodlands, M., & Wong, B. (1982). Comparability of self-concept among learning disabled, normal and gifted students. *Journal of Learning Disabilities, 15,* 470–475.

Wylie, R. (1974). *The self concept: A review of methodological considerations and measuring instruments.* Lincoln, NE: University of Nebraska Press.

6
The Minority in Person: Gifted Children in Therapy

In the four previous chapters, different sources of information have indicated that the majority of gifted children fare well socially. Yet many of the authors insist that a very sizeable minority of gifted children display pronounced social relations difficulties, although these authors would not dispute the foregoing conclusion about the "average" gifted child. This chapter is devoted to the minority of gifted children who do not fare well socially.

The size of the maladjusted minority is a matter of some dispute. Several researchers have in fact reported an incidence rate of severe social (Hitchfield cited in Janos, 1983) and psychiatric (Detzner & Schmidt, 1986) problems among gifted children that is lower than that of the population at large. However, some of the studies reviewed by Janos (1983), who focused on highly gifted rather than moderately gifted children, suggest that as many as 25% of that group are experiencing severe adjustment difficulties.

Let us assume that the gifted children experiencing social relations problems do in fact constitute a minority, but a minority large enough to merit special attention. This chapter begins with three case studies of gifted children seen in psychotherapy by the author. Following these case examples and an analysis of their common elements, suggestions are offered regarding the counseling of gifted children experiencing peer relations problems.

David, Age 14

David (names and biographical details have been changed) was brought to my office by his mother. In tears, she reported that his father wanted no involvement in David's psychological care and did not believe in psychologists. She said that the referral had been instigated by David's chemistry teacher, who described him as a walking "time bomb." David was reportedly disliked by everybody. When anyone at school attempted to talk to David about his problems, he would maintain that he did not have any.

David's mother was a social work assistant who had moved to Toronto from Vancouver 3 years prior to David's referral. She was of the *nisei* generation, born in Western Canada of Japanese parents. Her conversation was sprinkled with the jargon of psychological theories and therapies that Easterners stereotypically associate with the Pacific coast. Her primordial concern was David's happiness. She wanted him to "get in better touch with his feelings."

I met David's father several weeks later, when he came to drive David home from one of his therapy sessions. He asked to see me and spent most of the time making sure that I was familiar with all of David's mother's disordered features. The mother was described as a hysteric. There was no communication between the parents, but they had decided to stay together for the sake of David and his two younger brothers. David's father had no interest in marriage counseling. In his view, the difficulties at home were entirely attributable to his wife's pathology. David's father had immigrated from Japan. After a brilliant university career there, he worked as a researcher for a large company. He emphasized the fact that he wanted the road to success to be easier for David than it was for him. He also bemoaned the lack of discipline among today's young. Although achievement oriented and businesslike, David's father was much more easygoing than expected. Esteem for learning seemed prominent in his value system but only for reasons of career advancement.

David was attending a special school for talented science students. Although he recognized the need for therapy, he did not consider it a high priority and worried that the appointments would take too much time from his work. He had a friend who attended a workshop on time management conducted by a psychologist and asked if I could recommend some readings on time management. David acknowledged some difficulty in getting along with peers. In his opinion, they were picking on him because of his race. Thus, the problems were theirs, not his. Besides, he had no time for friends. David seemed rigid, hard-driven, and pressured.

David treated the therapy experience as he would a lesson in a required subject of moderate importance. He would carefully summarize each session (making the therapist's chore of preparing a progress note for his file unaccustomedly brief) and commit the main points to memory. Since there was no way of exorcising the scientific method from his thought process, I decided to make use of it. Together we reviewed journal articles on type A behavior and its consequences. David was initially more interested in the research designs and flaws in the logic than in the intended message. As a homework assignment, I instructed David to observe the social behavior of some high-achieving but socially successful classmate. David reported that this classmate was much more easygoing than him and slow to take offense. David remarked that this style would be much more "efficient."

At David's request, much of the therapy time was spent discussing his relationship with his parents. He respected his father but was quite distant from him. He deeply loved his mother but disobeyed her regularly and placed little credence in her advice. He and his mother were involved in frequent arguments. His mother would usually let him have his way to restore peace. In therapy, we explored alternate ways of responding to both parents. Because of the premature termination of treatment, I do not know if David ever implemented these.

One day, he arrived for his session and announced that he was changing his ways and becoming less driven and intense. Having understood the need for this, David had no time for any more therapy. His father called to thank me for the progress made.

Ellen, Age 15

Ellen was a student at a school that specialized in performing arts. She was referred by the guidance counselor, who felt that Ellen's impertinent attitude was affecting her academic progress. Most of her peers wanted little to do with her despite her musical and dramatic talents, attractive appearance, and winning smile. From her first therapy session on, Ellen attributed her difficulties to her parents' divorce. In a most histrionic way, she concluded that she was destined to forever experience emotional suffering because of her family's internal discord.

Ellen's allegiance wavered from one parent to the other. For the first few sessions, Ellen idolized her father and described her visits with him as her only respite from her Mom's domineering control and her peers' sarcasm. Her allegiance soon shifted as Dad's involvement with a new lady friend intensified. Ellen began to criticize her father. She felt that he had no more time for her and would offer her lavish gifts instead of affection and time. The exact pattern was then repeated with her mother, over a period of about 2 months. Ellen was able to see that she did not give either of her parent's new partners a chance to develop a relationship with her and that no prospective partner would likely meet her standards.

Ellen was shunned by most of her classmates, whom she regarded as unsophisticated. She had a small circle of close friends, who would gather, it seemed, to trade criticisms of teachers, parents, popular classmates, and each other. This subgroup was subject to much internal rivalry, inter-personal friction, and a series of vendettas. When Ellen clashed with the unproclaimed co-leader of this clique, she feigned indifference and defended herself well. She reserved expression of her profound and totally disproportionate anxiety and sorrow for her therapy session.

A major goal in therapy was to get her to see her parents, as well as teachers and peers, in a more balanced, objective way rather than in stark blacks and pure whites. As I got to know Ellen better and became more familiar with her parents during progress reviews, I realized that her special talents were not limited to music and drama. She knew people well. If overdramatized in their delivery, her criticisms of those around her always seemed to contain an uncanny element of truth. She was sensitive to the point of being an incessant gadfly; both peer and family relations were strained because of this.

While she was still in therapy, I happened to see Ellen performing in an experimental play. Her rendition of a homeless waif was flawless. She recognized me and came to the lobby to chat at intermission. I had difficulty containing her intrusive questions about my personal life and companions.

Ellen's therapy lasted most of a year. She was prone to bouts with depression, as well as elevated moods in which she became an almost totally saccharine Pollyanna, totally out of character. She enjoyed reviewing her life experiences, and she relished having someone listen to her criticisms of those around her. Her resistance to the necessary confronting communication was quite ephemeral. I consider her progress in therapy quite good.

Jeffrey, Age 8

Jeffrey was referred by his pediatrician. He was in a special class for young, gifted children, but was about to be asked to return to his home school because of incomplete written assignments, mumbling in class, and fights at recess. Psychoeducational appraisal indicated that Jeffrey might be considered both gifted and learning disabled. His motor speed and steadiness paled in contrast with his precocious language development and abstract reasoning skills. His written work was sloppy. I quizzed him on the content of one exercise sheet he was supposed to have completed in class. When he did not complete it in school, it was sent home as homework. He did not do it even then. His dislike of writing and defiance of authority were the prevailing themes in these exchanges. On a purely academic basis, it was clear that Jeffrey did not require any further drill on the content.

Jeffrey had been adopted when he was 4 months old. His parents feared that this caused the problem. They wanted to know if, in the course of his treatment, it was possible for Jeffrey to relive his infancy and "undo" the damage. They were also highly critical of the school system. They arrived at their first appointment armed with the rules and regulations regarding special education tribunals. They were certain that they would have to appeal an inappropriate school placement decision. In fact, they seemed to want to go through these proceedings as their contribution to systems change.

Jeffrey was involved in a type of activity therapy. Whenever the topic of peer relations was broached, he would avoid it. One day, he brought in a report card that lauded his potential but lambasted his work habits and behavior. When I asked if he wanted to discuss new ways of handling his peer relations, he looked at me sideways, as if to chide me for my naivete, and said to me, "You know, those things don't really change." He reluctantly agreed to discuss some alternatives anyway because "there's no harm in listening."

Both Jeffrey's parents were givers of advice. His father was a financial management consultant. His mother had opened a small, high-quality chocolate shop. This was a source of great pride. This shop was on a street of small stores and restaurants in a neighborhood where many students and young people lived. Her gregarious ways made it something of a "drop-in center" for neighboring merchants. Unfortunately, Jeffrey spent long periods of time supervised by his older sister while both parents worked. He did not get along with her. There were many family quarrels when the parents returned home to receive his sister's negative reports about his behavior.

Jeffrey was adamant that he did not have to obey his sister's directions. He had prepared a rather respectable legal argument. The Bible commands one to honor fathers and mothers only. There is a provincial law regarding following the directions of school authorities. There is nothing in law about big sisters. When Jeffrey informed his father of this, he was spanked, despite his mother's frenzied objections. He came to his next therapy session asking if it was possible to report a case of child abuse in the absence of any bruises or scars.

As I got to know Jeffrey better, I realized that he was totally unaware of the impact of his bossiness and stubbornness on his peer relations. In addition, he would often make unsolicited curt statements about the "way things are" to classmates who would argue back that things were not necessarily as Jeffrey saw them. Jeffrey's advice giving prematurely mirrored his parents vocation and avocation. The adversive effects of these behaviors were compounded by his whining, need for constant attention, and poor athletic ability. I felt that it was important for him to better appreciate the negative consequences of these behaviors. He reacted well to this and to my suggestion of practicing alternative behaviors on videotape. Despite Jeffrey's precocious learning ability, he was slow to acquire unfamiliar prosocial skills.

Common Elements

In all three cases, social problems did not emerge strictly out of giftedness. However, brightness and talent were interwoven into each of these youngsters' maladaptive behavior patterns. David was caught up in conflict between his parents and conflict between cultures and value systems. Membership in a racial minority may have exacerbated his problems. His obsessive character structure reflected his father's achievement values but might not have crystallized as much if he were not as successful in his studies and promising as a scientist.

Ellen's talents also figured in her difficulties, or, perhaps, were created by them. Her perceptiveness and expressiveness were put to good use on the stage, although they worked to her detriment in the arena of peer relations. Ellen's role in the family dynamics was probably more dysfunctional because of her keenness in sizing up people.

Jeffrey's displays of knowledge were also put to poor use in his attempts at relating with others. He was not really any more critical and defiant of authority than his parents. Whenever I looked at his sloppy schoolwork, I wondered whether his learning disability also contributed greatly to the difficult nature conveyed to others.

Thus, giftedness and other factors seemed to interact in the emergence of psychopathology. The complexity of such multiple etiologies, and the uniqueness of each case, have not been well captured in the empirical studies reviewed in the four previous chapters.

Counseling the Socially Maladjusted Gifted Child

Although there are many books that provide suggestions for the counseling of maladjusted gifted youth, there has been little systematic study of counseling strategies for this group. Hopefully, more research on intervention strategies for those gifted children who need it will emerge now that the question of *whether* they need it is largely resolved. The following sections are necessarily based on the author's experience rather than empirical investigation.

An Inevitable Tradeoff

When members of the minority of gifted children reach the stage of requiring special counseling, they often feel that they are rejected by their peers because of their special talents. This is sometimes expressed with anxiety and pain, sometimes with a pretended disdain of the majority's stereotyped banality. Rarely is there a recognition that they have any control over their peers' behavior.

In these situations, it is most useful to help gifted children wrestle with what appears to be an inevitable tradeoff. If they fail to learn the vernacular of the peer group, do not diversify their activities a bit, and express little interest in others, they will, quite logically, not achieve peer acceptance. The behavior of the peer group will be much more difficult to change than the gifted child's approach to them. The implication of the research summarized in the last four chapters is not that giftedness will automatically lead to a revered position on the highest rung of the social status ladder, but that giftedness will not be held against children socially in most situations.

Should they decide to diversify their activities and interests somewhat, they require the patience and support of adults, as well as the encouragement to not totally renounce all commitment to special areas of talent. Should they choose not to learn the ways of the majority, they may require some assistance from adults in locating a compatible group of exceptional peers. They can be helped to understand that, although there is a cost in terms of peer acceptance in the larger group, this does not have to be considered a catastrophe. Such interventions are sometimes helpful in sensitizing gifted children to this decision and making the consequences less painful whatever course they choose. Most importantly, the children must make this decision themselves; it cannot be imposed on them.

Social Problem Solving

Whatever the overall track record of social problem-solving techniques in enhancing children's social skills (Schneider & Byrne, 1985; Urbain & Kendall, 1980; Weissberg, 1985), these methods may have particular application to counseling the maladjusted minority among the gifted. Those with sharp social thinking skills may inherently reject being directly and uncritically told what to do. There are few important social behaviors that are totally without disadvantages. Many bright children are quick to perceive the shortcomings of any panacea presented with oversimplified justification. However, they can be helped to appreciate their alternatives, contemplate the implications of each, and decide on action strategies. This mode of intervention is perhaps more appropriate to the socially intelligent than to any other segment of the population at large.

"You Should Know Better"

Bright children resent, perhaps more than anything else, any insinuation that there are separate standards of social behavior for gifted children. Perhaps they should indeed be expected to display more mature social behavior because of their repertoire of social knowledge and ability to understand social consequences. However, they object strenuously to more stringent expectations being mandatory. Adult attempts to change the behavior of gifted children by means of appeals to their brightness are likely to backfire.

Many bright children are perceptive and critical in social situations. They may think things through and harbor a degree of not always unhealthy skepticism. This can be seen as a negative attitude toward the peer group, school, community, or family. At times, they can in fact manifest a negative attitude. Many adults instinctively intervene by telling bright children to change their attitudes. This is an ineffective strategy. Few children turn their attitudes on an off like electrical applicances. They are more likely to change their behavior than their thinking in response to an adult's brief remarks.

As discussed in Chapter 5, some gifted children have been found to be hypersensitive in social situations. This does not mean that it would be healthy to handle them always with kid gloves. However, there are some implications for adult–child relations. In particular, they typically react best to private discussions about their behavior where necessary, reassured that the conversation will not affect their reputations among peers.

Determining the Locus of Intervention

Sometimes gifted children who are referred for counseling are reacting to unfavorable educational surroundings, unsympathetic communities, or unstimulating programs. Counseling can sometimes help these youngsters cope with less than optimal environments if no environmental change is possible. However, it is imperative to make the effort to improve their situations. The impact of schools on the social development of the gifted is the subject of the next chapter.

References

Detzner, M., & Schmidt, M.H. (1986). Are highly gifted children and adolescents especially susceptible to anorexia nervosa? In K.A. Heller & J.M. Feldhusen (Eds.), *Identifying and nurturing the gifted* (pp. 149–162). Toronto: Huber.

Janos, P.M. (1983). *The psychological vulnerabilites of children of very superior intellectual ability*. Doctoral dissertation. Ohio State University. (University Microfilms No. 83-18, 377)

Schneider, B.H., & Byrne, B.M. (1985). Children's social skills training: A meta-analysis. In B.H. Schneider, K.H. Rubin, & J.E. Ledingham (Eds.), *Children's peer relations: Issues in assessment and intervention* (pp. 175–192). New York: Springer-Verlag.

Urbain, E.S., & Kendall, P.C. (1980). Review of social-cognitive problem-solving interventions with children. *Psychological Bulletin, 8,* 109–143.

Weissberg, R.P. (1985). Problem-solving programs for the classroom. In B.H. Schneider, K. Rubin, & J.E. Ledingham (Eds.), *Children's peer relations: Issues in assessment and intervention* (pp. 225–242). New York: Springer-Verlag.

7
School Life and the Social Development of the Gifted

There are four types of students: (1) Those who absorb everything they hear like a sponge; (2) Those who, like a funnel, receive at one end and dismiss at another; (3) Those who, like a strainer, allow the wine to flow out and retain the lees; (4) Those who, like a sieve, separate the bran from the fine flour. It is the task of parents and teachers to teach each child in accordance with his own way. (From *Ethics of the Fathers*, quoted by Matzner-Beckerman 1984)

Not long after the advent of free compulsory public education in North America, Yoder (1894) bemoaned the fact that there is no institution that can more rapidly and effectively stifle precocious intellect and creativity than the public school. Similar laments can be overheard to this day at gatherings of the parents of gifted children. Few issues can arouse more passion than the question of what type of education is best for the young gifted in our midst.

There are a number of viable alternatives in educational programming for the gifted. Each of these alternatives has possible ramifications for the peer relations of participants as well as for their cognitive growth. The most traditional approach, although not without some contemporary adherents, is acceleration, allowing gifted children to "skip" grades until they reach a level commensurate with their knowledge and capacities. The obvious drawback in terms of peer relations is the fact that the acceleraters will be younger than their classmates. Furthermore, they will *always* be younger than their classmates, barring the unlikely possibility that they will at some point be asked to repeat a school year to bring them back to the age range of their peers. Thus, even if an accelerated 9 year old appears to interact well with classmates who are 10 or 11, it cannot be assumed that the same child 5 years later will be socially compatible with 15 and 16 year olds. Nevertheless, there are many case studies of successful acceleration, starting with the Terman classics (Terman, 1925; see Chapters 1 and 4).

Varieties of special education programs for the gifted continue to proliferate as awareness of the need increases. A major advantage of special enrichment is that the pupil remains associated with age-compatible classmates. Presumably, the curriculum is *qualitatively* as well as *quantitatively* different from that of the regular class; this may not really be the case if the child is placed one grade higher. Furthermore, the special enrichment programs also bring gifted children into contact with each other; acceleration does not necessarily accomplish this. Association with gifted peers may bring not only enhanced intellectual stimulation but also social support.

As with special education programs for all other types of exceptional children, there is considerable controversy as to whether special programming for the gifted should be delivered in special classes for the gifted, or on a part-time basis to gifted children who remain in regular classes and schools. In addition to the possible impact on the children's social development, which will be considered in the following discussion, there are obvious ramifications for the children's academic programming. A 3-hour/week enrichment program can only be successful if measures are taken to ensure that the remaining 27 or so hours of the school week are educationally beneficial to the gifted participants.

How might part-time enrichment affect the peer relations of gifted children? Obviously, the gifted children remain in interaction with nongifted peers. As detailed in Chapter 2, this cannot be considered an inherent drawback; we cannot assume that they will be rejected. Some sort of identification or labeling process will likely take place, and the child's peers will be well aware of the participants' designation as gifted. The peer group will be reminded of the participants' gifted status at least once a week when the participants in the special program are withdrawn. At first glance, one might consider any such labeling as harmful and predict that it would lead to peer rejection. Indeed, many parents intuitively object to their children being "singled out" for any type of special school treatment. While the peer group will be acutely aware of the child's participation in part-time enrichment, there is little basis for any presupposition that the peers' reaction will be negative. Robinson (1986) pointed out that the gifted are labeled because they deviate from the norm in a positive way. Reviewing the literature on attitudes within the school system toward the label "gifted," she concluded that the few studies that have been conducted on the impact of the gifted label have yielded contradictory findings. Pending further research, mention might be made of enrichment activities available outside of school in some communities. These do not involve the child being labeled at all within the school. Often operated by universities, museums, and advocacy groups for the gifted, these may include summer camps and Saturday morning enrichment programs.

The final major educational alternative for the gifted is the establishment of special classes or schools. These do have the distinct pedagogical advantage of permitting the development of a curriculum exclusively for the gifted. To the degree that such curricula are well designed and properly executed, they ensure that school time will be intellectually productive for the gifted; acceleration and part-time enrichment offer no such guarantee. The implications in terms of peer relations are drastic. The gifted child in a full-time special program is essentially removed from social contact with nongifted peers. This in itself is only an advantage if the gifted child has been rejected by them. As detailed in Chapter 2, this should not be assumed to apply to the majority of gifted children. On the other hand, such separation from the normal peer group may deprive the gifted of the opportunity to master the social skills needed to relate to the nongifted majority. In place of a "normal" peer group, the child's gifted peers serve as companions and sources of social validation. This may allow for mutual support, encouragement of each other's special interests, cross-fertilization of more advanced "social intelligence," and more appropriate role modeling. On the other hand, distance from "normal" peers may have a price. If, as discussed in Chapter 5, gifted children have difficulty receiving messages that indicate that they are *not* disliked, segregation from regular class peers can only aggravate this problem, for they will be only more cut off from such signals. In fact, a wide range of unhealthy stereotypes about "normal" people might emerge among the special class participants. Moreover, special class or special school placement may also result in enhanced competition. Intensified pressures to achieve may leave little time for social life. A self-presentation characterized by anxiety, stress and hurry may be introduced into the pupil's social relationships.

Evaluating the Impact of School Programming

Designing research to evaluate the impact of school programs on the social development of the gifted is certainly no easier than designing any other research reviewed in this book. A number of salient issues emerge. Ideally, one would like to know not only how children change after programing has been introduced, but how they would have changed and developed in the absence of the program. This entails the use of experimental designs involving control groups. Only the most patient and scientifically informed of parents would allow their children to be placed in a control group of this kind. In some jurisdictions, e.g., the province of Ontario, it is compulsory by law for school districts to provide suitable special programs for all exceptional children, including the gifted. Thus, a traditional, controlled study might even be illegal. The same applies to time-series designs, in which children's development during a time period in which they receive programming is compared with their development during periods of time during which no programming is delivered. This would be impossible because practical and legal if not ethical conditions preclude there being a period of time with no special programming.

Even if one were able to conduct an experimental study with some sort of control group or condition, it would be important to ensure that the control group children are equivalent to those in the special program. This is best accomplished by random assignment of subjects to groups, which is, again, highly problematic. However, it is otherwise very difficult to establish that the children receiving the program started out with social and intellectual development equivalent to that of controls.

The next design consideration is the selection of outcome measures. Should a program be evaluated on the basis of goals it seeks to achieve? Or should any program for the gifted automatically be judged according to certain prespecified criteria? Are changes in academic achievement, creativity, social skills, and self-concept relevant to the evaluation? If so, how should these be weighted and compared? Is any program that enhances self-concept valuable, even if the children do not learn a great deal? Or is any increment in creativity to be considered an important accomplishment, even if peer relations seem to suffer? These crucial questions find answers only in the values of the researchers and the communities in which they work.

Today's accountability-hungry taxpayer may dictate that a program be evaluated soon after it is introduced. However, many programs may improve after they have been first implemented. Staff members become more familiar with the gifted children and their needs. "Wrinkles" may be ironed out and selection procedures refined. Unfortunately, most programs are evaluated very soon after their introduction. There are very few follow-up studies that investigate the long-term impact of special programs on the social development of the gifted. As with any other type of program evaluation, the researcher and participants may be concerned that the program might be discontinued if it turns out not to fully accomplish its mission. This may affect participation in the study and color the interpretation of the findings.

Research on the Impact of Schools

A summary of known studies on the impact of school programs on the social development of gifted youngsters appears in Table 7.1. As indicated, there have been a number of studies conducted with the various modalities of school interventions previously discussed. Gifted children of all ages have participated.

Fortunately, this literature contains several experimental studies in which it was possible to randomly assign subjects to intervention and control groups. The results of some of the quasi-experimental studies are of much less value because possible preexisting differences between the special program and comparison groups may have attenuated the findings. For example, several investigators compared the group of children who

TABLE 7.1. Studies evaluating impact of special programming on social development of the gifted.

Author and date	Age	Type of program	Design	Outcome measure	Results
Goldworth (1959)	Grades 4–8	Enrichment 3 hr/week	Experimental	Peer nominations	NS
Gallagher, Greenman, Karnes, & King (1960)	Grades 2–3	Modifications of regular classroom programs	Pre- and postcomparison	Peer nominations	–
Lutfiyya (1977/1978)	Grades 4–12	Part-time enrichment	Quasi-experimental	Self-concept	NS
Maugh (1977)	Grades 3–6	Part-time enrichment	Quasi-experimental	Self-concept	NS[a]
Carter (1978)	Grades 7–11	?	Ex post facto	Self-concept	+
Lytle & Campbell (1979/1980)	Grade 4	Enrichment 2 hr/week	Quasi-experimental	Peer nominations	NS
Rodgers (1979/1980)	Elementary	Enrichment 1 day/week	Experimental	Self-concept	NS
Fults (1980/1981)	Grades 4–6	Part-time enrichment	Pre- and postcomparison	Self-concept	–
Coleman & Fults (1982)	Grades 4–6	Enrichment 1 day/week	Quasi-experimental	Self-concept	–
Evans & Marken (1982)	Grades 6–8	Full-time special class	Ex post facto	Self-concept	NS
Maddux, Scheiber, & Bass (1982)	Grades 5–6	Full-time special class	Quasi-experimental	Self-concept	NS
		Enrichment 3 hr/week		Peer ratings	–[b]
Miller (1982)	Grades 9–12	Part-time enrichment	Ex post facto	Self-concept	NS
Pollin (1983)	Grades 7–8	Accelerated grade placement	Quasi-experimental	Self-report scales	NS
Kolloff & Feldhusen (1984)	Grades 3–6	Enrichment 2 hr/week	Experimental	Self-concept	NS
Schneider, Clegg, Byrne, Ledingham, & Crombie (1986)	Grades 5 and 8	Full-time special class	Ex post facto	Academic self-concept	–
				Social self-concept	NS
				Physical self-concept	NS

Note. + = improvement for special program group. – = deterioration for special program group. NS = no significant change.
[a] Significant improvement at ninth-grade level only.
[b] Significant deterioration in peer esteem for fifth graders in full-time program only.

received special programming with a group of children who had been referred to the program but were not selected or did not meet the admission criteria (e.g., Coleman & Fults, 1982; Lytle & Campbell, 1979). Since these children were from the outset different from those in the programs, the comparison data are difficult to interpret.

One study of particular interest was conducted by Maddux et al. (1982). This study compared the effects of part-time enrichment with those of full-time special class placement. This study is valuable because it encompassed both major modalities of enrichment programming. Although the subjects were not randomly assigned to intervention and control groups, an appropriate comparison group of gifted children was used. Tests were conducted to establish that there were no preexisting differences between the experimental and comparison groups on several salient dimensions. Maddux and co-workers found no differences among the groups in terms of self-concept. However, in one of the two grades studied, gifted youngsters in the full-time program suffered a deterioration in peer acceptance.

These findings are consistent with the general trend of this literature. Most of the studies in Table 7.1 indicate either no significant change in social development or significant deterioration in social development as a result of special programming for the gifted. These disappointing conclusions appear to apply across age ranges, in a variety of locations, to several different indices of social competence, in studies that utilized a variety of different research designs. The results are underscored by a particularly interesting follow-up component in the study by Coleman and Fults (1982). They actually found that when students *left* a special program for the gifted, their self-concepts became more positive.

There are a number of possible explanations for the findings. In the introductions to several of the studies, the authors speculate that the gifted youngsters may be rejected socially in their regular programs. If this were the case, special programming and association with gifted peers would enhance their social acceptance. However, as previously noted, this hypothesis is questionable, as wholesale peer rejection of the gifted has not been found in most studies.

Second, entrance into a special program means that the gifted children who are accustomed to being the intellectual leaders of their hetero-geneous peer groups are placed in the company of peers who are their intellectual equals or superiors. Social comparison theory (Bandura, 1971) suggests that individuals evaluate themselves in reference to those who immediately surround them. Thus, the self-concept of a gifted child who was previously "a big fish in a small pond" may understandably diminish upon entrance to a special class (see Coleman & Fults, 1982, for fuller discussion).

Twelve of the studies of school program effects summarized in Table 7.1 utilized self-concept as an outcome measure. Only the study by Schneider et al. (1986) reported self-concept results differentiated by self-concept domain, though reanalysis of the original data in several of the other studies would also permit domain-specific inferences. The results of this study should be interpreted with considerable caution because of the *ex post facto* design. The participants in the special class group and integrated gifted control group were not randomly assigned. The controls were gifted youngsters in a neighboring school district, which at the time of the study, did not have segregated special classes for the gifted. These two groups did not differ significantly in terms of age, sex, or IQ. Unfortunately, there were no data available regarding the self-concepts of the gifted children in special classes prior to their admission to special classes. Nevertheless, the results of this study are of some interest despite the *ex post facto* design, because they indicate that while the special class group scored lower than the integrated gifted controls on self-concept, this was limited to academic self-concept. There were no significant differences between the groups in terms of social or physical self-concept. Thus, the results of Schneider and his colleagues fit well with social comparison theory, in that the self-concepts of the gifted children in special classes reflect the heightened academic competence of those around them.

Further investigation of the impact of special programs on the various facets of self-esteem is clearly needed and warranted. If it emerges that the "damage" caused by special programs to the self-concept of the gifted is restricted to the academic domain, this entire body of literature may come to be reinterpreted in a much more positive light. Even if special programming does exact a toll on the social development of participants, the nature and extent of the possible damage is not easily discernible from the studies. First of all, we need to establish whether the findings indicate that previously well-adjusted participants became maladjusted and rejected once placed in special programs. If this is the case, the findings are of dramatic concern and indicate some need for change in special programs or in selection criteria. However, a systematic decrement limited to academic self-concept from the highest levels to the middle of the scale would provide little cause for alarm. Although Blatz's (1966) views may (and did) sound heretical to some educators and psychologists, he emphasized the importance of what he called constructive experiences of failure in helping the child learn and grow. Special programs may provide such constructive experiences of failure, perhaps sorely needed by students who were not previously challenged in school.

Some research has established that when special programming for the gifted is introduced, two parallel social systems begin to operate. The gifted children associate with other special program participants; the nongifted no longer include the special program participants in their friendship choices (Mann, 1957). The interpretation of this finding is heavily value laden. It is desirable for gifted children to associate with each other, providing intellectual stimulation as well as support and encouragement for their individual pursuits. However, it may be seen as negative if the gifted associate only with the gifted because of lack of ability or desire to relate with nongifted peers. In addition, if these two systems emerge because the gifted are rejected for reasons of their special program status, these results cannot be considered a positive development.

Enhancing the Impact of Special Programs

Of course, the studies reviewed here have evaluated the impact of programs as we now know them on the social relations of the gifted, not the impact of programs as they might optimally be implemented. A number of changes in certain prevailing program features might considerably alter this picture. As noted by Janos and Robinson (1985), there has been no research to determine what specific variables in school programming for the gifted are associated with successful outcome. The following speculative suggestions for improvement are offered in the absence of a relevant data base.

First of all, the appeal of special programs to gifted children who now shun them might be enhanced. It is a tragic fact that large numbers of gifted children choose not to participate in special programs for the gifted even when they have the opportunity to do so. In fact, such youngsters are so numerous that they have been used as control groups with which special program participants have been compared (e.g., Miller, 1982). One might speculate that these nonparticipants are gifted children who are more socially than academically oriented. If so, they might provide more optimal models of social competence within the gifted programs. Such pupils might be attracted by measures that ensure that their grades will not suffer because of their participation in special programming. Such measures are already operational in some enrichment programs.

Young, Gifted, and Hurried

Rapid academic advancement is something of a tradition in gifted education. The first special classes for the gifted in the New York City public schools were in fact referred to as rapid advancement programs (Fox & Washington, 1985), or "the rapids." In times of economic depression and war, the advantages of this approach would probably outweigh any costs in the area of social development. However, at this point, the personal and social impact of the work pressure often placed on the gifted student in special programs might be carefully reevaluated. Enrichment programs should differ from regular classes in terms of the cognitive complexity of what is taught, the opportunities for creative thinking and the pursuit of individual areas of talent. This does not mean that the students' academic assignments must be so lengthy that the gifted have no time to explore nonacademic aspects of their youth. Although there is a certain seductive appeal in enabling students to complete university-level courses while in high school, or to amass credits sooner, we must realize that abbreviating the childhoods of the gifted may not be without cost. Furthermore, giving gifted youngsters more work to do in the same amount of time as other pupils may actually interfere with the provision of an enriched learning environment. In one Canadian high school, many of the most capable students are invited to participate in an annual exchange program in Europe. Those in the special program for the gifted are not permitted to participate because this would mean taking too much time from their studies! Of all the students in that school, only the gifted are deprived of perhaps the school's best opportunities for enhancing social and cultural maturity, not to mention the opportunities for *in vivo* lessons in geography, history, foreign languages, and social skills.

Finally, special programs could increasingly emphasize social interaction in general, and specifically the interaction of gifted and nongifted youngsters. While there is a viable argument in favor of special classes for some gifted youngsters, there is little justification for a gifted youngster being entirely deprived of contact with nongifted peers. The gifted may be able to serve as a resource to other youngsters. Peer tutoring is one of the most effective forms of academic remediation (see review by Gauthier, Loranger, & Ladouceur, 1984). This learning experience can consolidate the gifted pupils' understanding of subject matter; only if one understands something thoroughly can one explain it to someone else. Furthermore, this social interchange can alter the perception of the gifted by their nongifted counterparts and vice versa.

Modeling Effects

Many authors have stressed the impact of adult mentors on gifted youth and vividly described educational gains that emerge within the context of these relationships (Levinson, Darrow, Klein, Levinson, & McKee, 1978). There also has been some study of the characteristics of effective classroom teachers of the gifted. The most systematic research in this area was conducted by Bishop (1981). He completed an extensive study of 109 Georgia school teachers who were nominated as excellent by gifted pupils. These teachers differed from the average classroom teacher in a number of ways. They had higher IQs, pronounced literary and artistic interests, high needs for achievement, and a student-centered orientation. Unfortunately, Bishop did not study the social competence of these outstanding educators. Given the apparent major influence of adult role models on the learning, motivation, and personal adjustment of gifted children, this area may be worthy of some attention. Maddux, Samples-Lachmann, and Cummings (1985) found that gifted Texas junior high school students prefer teachers with personal-social strengths over those who emphasize the cognitive or classroom management aspects of teaching (although contradictory findings were reported by Milgram [1979] in a study conducted with gifted children in Israel). Mentors and teachers of bright children might be recruited from among the socially gifted if it emerges that they are not already well represented in those roles.

The Case for Allocating Resources to the Gifted

This book might have provided more ammunition to those who promote special programs for the gifted if it had been able to portray giftedness as a natural resource in imminent danger of depletion by means of the incessant attacks of hostile childhood peers. However, the data are not consistent with such an image. Insensitivity to, and outright rejection of, young gifted peers are not unknown. However, such treatment cannot be seen as the prevalent state of affairs. Thus, one cannot argue for special programming for the gifted on that basis. The compelling argument for special programs for gifted children is the need to stimulate and cultivate their intellectual, creative, motivational, artistic, and scientific talents.

My values will not permit closing with the threat that if we do not cultivate the talents of the gifted, we will be deprived of their contributions to society in later life. Rather, I will close with a reminder that the failure to adequately stimulate the intellect of any child—gifted, retarded, learning disabled, or "normal"—is one of the cruelest blows any society can inflict upon its young.

References

Bandura, A. (1971). Vicarious and self-reinforcement processes. In R. Glaser (Ed.), *The nature of reinforcement.* Orlando, FL: Academic Press.

Bishop, W. (1981). Characteristics of teachers judged successfully intellectually gifted by high achieving high school students. In W. Barbe & J. Renzulli (Eds.), *Psychology and education of the gifted* (pp. 422–432). New York: Irvington.

Blatz, W.E. (1966). *Human security: Some reflections.* Toronto: University of Toronto Press.

Carter, F. (1978). The relationship of gifted adolescents self-concept to achievement, sex, grade level, and membership in a self-contained academic program for the gifted. *Dissertation Abstracts International, 39,* 1406A. (University Microfilms No. 7815954).

Coleman, J., & Fults, B. (1982). Self-concept and the gifted classroom: The role of social comparisons. *Gifted Child Quarterly, 26,* 116–120.

Evans, E., & Marken, D. (1982). Multiple outcome assessment of special class placement for gifted students: A comparative study. *Gifted Child Quarterly, 26,* 126–132.

Fox, L.H., & Washington, J. (1985). Programs for the gifted and talented: Past, present and future. In F.D. Horowitz & M. O'Brian (Eds.), *The gifted and talented: Developmental perspectives* (pp. 197–222). Washington, DC: American Psychological Association.

Fults, E.A. (1980/1981). The effect of an instructional program on the creative thinking skills, self-concept and leadership of intellectually and academically gifted elementary students. *Dissertation Abstracts International, 41,* 2931A. (University Microfilms No. 80-29001).

Gallagher, J.J., Greenman, M., Karnes, M., & King, A. (1960). Individual classroom adjustments for gifted children in elementary schools. *Exceptional Children, 26,* 409–422.

Gauthier, D., Loranger, M., & Ladouceur, R. (1984). Le renfocement des comportements académiques: Une stratégie économique dans l'intervention en milieu scolaire. *Canadian Psychology, 25,* 14–22.

Goldworth, M. (1959). The effects of an elementary school fast-learner program on children's social relationships. *Exceptional Children, 26,* 59–63.

Janos, P.M., & Robinson, N.M. (1985). Psychosocial development in intellectually gifted children. In F. Horowitz & M. O'Brien (Eds.), *The gifted and talented: Developmental perspectives* (pp. 149–196). Washington, DC: American Psychological Association.

Kolloff, M.B., & Feldhusen, J.F. (1984). The effects of enrichment of self-concept and creative thinking. *Gifted Child Quarterly, 28,* 53–57.

Levinson, D.J., Darrow, C.M., Klein, E.B., Levinson, M.H., & McKee, B. (1978). Psychological development. In D.F. Ricks, A. Thomas, & M. Roff (Eds.), *Life history research* (Vol. 3, pp. 243–258). Minneapolis: University of Minnesota Press.

Lutfiyya, L.A. (1977/1978). A comparison of the achievement, self-concept, creative thinking and realistic self-evaluation of gifted and talented students within and without special programs for gifted and talented students in grades 4–12. *Dissertation Abstracts International, 38,* 5382A. (University Microfilms No. 7801162).

Lytle, W., & Campbell, N. (1979). Do special programs affect the social status of the gifted? *Elementary School Journal, 80,* 93–97.

Maddux, C.D., Samples-Lachmann, I., & Cummings, R. (1985). Preferences of gifted students for selected teachers characteristics. *Gifted Child Quarterly, 29,* 160–163.

Maddux, C.D., Scheiber, L., & Bass, J. (1982). Self-concept and social distance in gifted children. *Gifted Child Quarterly, 26,* 77–81.

Mann, H. (1957). How real are friendships of gifted and typical children in a program of partial segregation? *Exceptional Children, 23,* 199–206.

Matzner-Beckerman, S. (1984). *The Jewish child: Halakhic perspectives.* New York: Ktav.

Maugh, V.M. (1977). An analysis of attitudes of selected academically talented elementary school students toward self-concept and school and of selected elementary teachers toward the academically talented student. (Doctoral dissertation, University of Southern Mississippi, 1977). *Dissertation Abstracts International, 38,* 2458A) (University Microfilms No. 77-22880).

Milgram, R.M. (1979). Perception of teacher behavior in gifted and nongifted children. *Journal of Educational Psychology, 71,* 125–128.

Miller, W.E. (1982/1983). A comparative analysis of segregated versus non-segregated educational programming for gifted students in self-concepts and selected other variables. (Doctoral dissertation, Pennsylvania State University, 1982/1983). *Dissertation Abstracts International, 43,* 8228A. (University Microfilms No. 82285).

Pollin, L. (1983). The effects of acceleration on the social and emotional development of gifted students. In C. Benbow & J. Stanley (Eds.), *Academic precocity: Aspects of its development* (pp. 160–179). Baltimore: Johns Hopkins University Press.

Robinson, A. (1986). The identification and labeling of gifted children: What does research tell us? In K.A. Heller and J.F. Feldhusen (Eds.), *Identifying and nurturing the gifted* (pp. 103–110). Toronto: Huber.

Rodgers, B.S. (1979/1980). Effects of an enrichment program screening process on the self-concept and others-concept of gifted elementary children. (Doctoral dissertation, University of Cincinnati, 1979/1980). *Dissertation Abstracts International, 41,* 3906A–3097A. (University Microfilms No. 80-02135).

Schneider, B.H., Clegg, M.R., Byrne, B.M., Ledingham, J.E., & Crombie, G. (1986). *The social consequences of giftedness in Ontario schools.* Unpublished research report, Social Sciences and Humanities Research Council of Canada and Ontario Ministry of Education.

Terman, L.M. (1925). *Genetic studies of genius.* Stanford: Stanford University Press.

Yoder, A. (1894). Study of the boyhoods of great men. *Pedagogical Seminary, 3,* 134–156.

Author Index

Subject Index